Fertility and Reproduction

Series Editor: Cara Acred

Volume 247

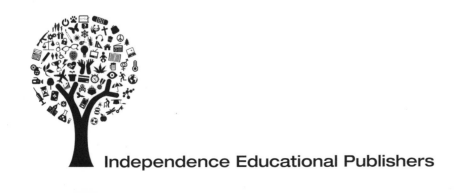

Independence Educational Publishers

First published by Independence Educational Publishers

The Studio, High Green

Great Shelford

Cambridge CB22 5EG

England

© Independence 2013

Copyright

Photocopy licence

British Library Cataloguing in Publication Data

Fertility and reproduction. -- (Issues ; 247)
1. Human reproductive technology--Moral and ethical
aspects.
I. Series II. Acred, Cara editor of compilation.
176-dc23

ISBN-13: 978 1 86168 649 7

Printed in Great Britain

MWL Print Group Ltd

Contents

Chapter 1: Infertility, IVF and alternatives

Chapter 2: Reproductive ethics

Introduction

Fertility and Reproduction is Volume 247 in the **ISSUES** series. The aim of the series is to offer current, diverse information about important issues in our world, from a UK perspective.

ABOUT FERTILITY AND REPRODUCTION

As many as one in seven couples can have problems conceiving a baby. There are many reasons for infertility and, today, many different solutions. IVF is one of the most widely known fertility treatments on the market, but to whom should it be made available is a hotly debated topic. When it comes to being a parent, how old is too old? This book explores the ethical and scientific issues surrounding infertility, presenting opinions on challenging concepts such as 'saviour siblings' and sex selection, as well as considering the processes of adoption and surrogacy.

OUR SOURCES

Titles in the **Issues** series are designed to function as educational resource books, providing a balanced overview of a specific subject.

The information in our books is comprised of facts, articles and opinions from many different sources, including:

- Newspaper reports and opinion pieces
- Website factsheets
- Magazine and journal articles
- Statistics and surveys
- Government reports
- Literature from special interest groups

A NOTE ON CRITICAL EVALUATION

Because the information reprinted here is from a number of different sources, readers should bear in mind the origin of the text and whether the source is likely to have a particular bias when presenting information (or when conducting their research). It is hoped that, as you read about the many aspects of the issues explored in this book, you will critically evaluate the information presented.

It is important that you decide whether you are being presented with facts or opinions. Does the writer give a biased or unbiased report? If an opinion is being expressed, do you agree with the writer? Is there potential bias to the 'facts' or statistics behind an article?

ASSIGNMENTS

In the back of this book, you will find a selection of assignments designed to help you engage with the articles you have been reading and to explore your own opinions. Some tasks will take longer than others and there is a mixture of design, writing and research-based activities that you can complete alone or in a group.

FURTHER RESEARCH

At the end of each article we have listed its source and a website that you can visit if you would like to conduct your own research. Please remember to critically evaluate any sources that you consult and consider whether the information you are viewing is accurate and unbiased.

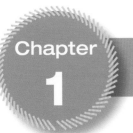

Infertility, IVF and alternatives

Infertility – a basic understanding

About one in seven couples can have some problems conceiving a baby. However, over nine in ten couples having regular sex will conceive within two years. There are various causes of subfertility, both in men and in women. However, there will be no reason found for the subfertility in about three in ten cases. Some reasons are easier to treat than others.

What is infertility?

Infertility means difficulty in conceiving (becoming pregnant) despite having regular sex when not using contraception. There is no definite cut-off point to say when a couple is infertile. Many couples take several months to conceive. About 84 couples out of 100 conceive within a year of trying. About 92 couples out of 100 conceive within two years. Looking at this another way, about one in seven couples do not conceive within a year of trying. However, more than half of these couples will conceive over the next year, without any treatment.

Doctors usually say that a couple is infertile if they have not conceived in two years, despite regular sexual intercourse.

It is usually worth seeing a GP if you have not conceived after one year of trying. A GP can check for some common causes, talk things over, and discuss possible options. You may want to see your GP earlier, if the woman in the couple is over the age of 35 or if either partner has a history of fertility problems.

A quick review of how pregnancy occurs

To conceive, an egg (ovum) from the woman has to combine with a sperm from the man. An ovum is released from an ovary when a woman ovulates. This usually occurs once a month between 12 and 16 days from the start of your last period if you have a regular monthly cycle of 28–30 days. The ovum travels down a Fallopian tube to the middle of the womb (uterus) over 12–24 hours.

Sperm lie next to the cervix (neck of the womb) when a man ejaculates (comes) during sex. The sperm travel up past the cervix to get into the main part of the uterus, and into the Fallopian tubes. If there are sperm in the Fallopian tubes then one may combine with (fertilise) the ovum to make an embryo. The tiny embryo travels down into the uterus and attaches to the lining of the uterus. The embryo then grows and matures into a baby.

What can cause fertility problems?

Ovulation problems in women

Not ovulating is the cause of problems in about three in ten couples. In some women this is a permanent problem. In some it is intermittent: some months ovulation occurs, and some months it doesn't. There are various causes of ovulation problems including:

⇨ Early (premature) menopause.

⇨ Polycystic ovary syndrome (PCOS). This can also cause excessive hair growth, acne, and menstrual problems, and is associated with obesity.

⇨ Hormone problems – for example, too much prolactin hormone. This hormone is produced by the pituitary gland that lies just beneath the brain and helps with milk production. Too little or too much thyroxine hormone (produced by the thyroid gland in the neck) also affects fertility.

⇨ Being very underweight or overweight. This can affect your hormone balance which can affect ovulation. In particular, women with anorexia nervosa often do not ovulate.

⇨ Excessive exercise (such as regular long-distance running) can affect your hormone balance ,which can affect ovulation.

⇨ Chronic (long-term) illnesses. Some women with severe chronic illnesses, such as uncontrolled diabetes, cancers and kidney failure, may not ovulate.

⇨ A side-effect from some medicines is a rare cause. Medicines that sometimes cause this include anti-inflammatory painkillers and some chemotherapy medicines. Some street drugs such as cannabis and cocaine can also affect your ability to ovulate.

⇨ Various other problems with the ovary such as certain genetic problems.

Fallopian tube, cervix or uterine problems

These are the cause in about two in ten couples with infertility. Problems include:

⇨ Endometriosis, which causes about one in 20 cases of infertility. Tissue that normally lines the uterus (endometrium) is found outside of the uterus. It is trapped in the pelvic area and can affect the ovaries, uterus and nearby structures. It often causes lower abdominal pain and/or painful periods.

⇨ Previous infection of the uterus and fallopian tubes (pelvic inflammatory disease (PID)) is another common cause. Chlamydial infection can be a cause of PID. PID can cause scarring and damage which can affect fertility. For example, scar tissue may block the egg (ovum) from travelling down the fallopian tubes.

⇨ Previous surgery to the fallopian tubes, cervix or uterus.

⇨ Large fibroids, which may also cause problems, although this is debated by some experts. A fibroid is a benign (non-cancerous) growth of the uterus (womb).

Male problems

These occur in about two in ten cases. Some men are born with testes that do not make any sperm or they make very few sperm. Some are born without testes or without a vas deferens.

The most common reason for male infertility is a problem with sperm due to an unknown cause. The sperm may be reduced in number, less mobile (less able to swim forwards), and/or be abnormal in their form.

There are a variety of things that may affect sperm production and male infertility. These include:

⇨ Certain hormone problems.

⇨ Current or past infection of the testes.

⇨ Tumours of the testes.

⇨ Testes that haven't descended (dropped) properly.

⇨ Side-effects of some medicines and street drugs. These include: sulfasalazine, nitrofurantoin, tetracyclines, cimetidine, colchicine, allopurinol, some chemotherapy drugs, cannabis, cocaine and anabolic steroids.

⇨ Regular excess heat (regular saunas, hot baths, etc.) is possibly a cause.

⇨ Environmental factors may be relevant in some men. For example, a lot of exposure to chemicals, X-rays or heavy metals.

⇨ A varicocele may possibly affect male fertility. A varicocele is common and is like a varicose vein in the scrotum (the skin that covers the testes). Varicoceles are found in just over one in ten men with normal sperm and one in four men with abnormal sperm.

Age can be a factor

⇨ Older women tend to be less fertile than younger women. The fall-off of fertility seems to be greatest once you are past your middle 30s. For women aged 35–39, the chance of conceiving is about half that of women aged 19–26. It is also thought that men over the age of 35 are half as likely to achieve a pregnancy when compared with men younger than 25.

Some general advice

The chance of conceiving gradually goes down over time. However, for couples where no cause is found for the problem, there is still a good chance of conceiving without treatment. In such couples, without treatment:

⇨ About half who do not conceive within one year conceive within the next year.

⇨ Those who do not conceive within three years still have about a one in four chance of

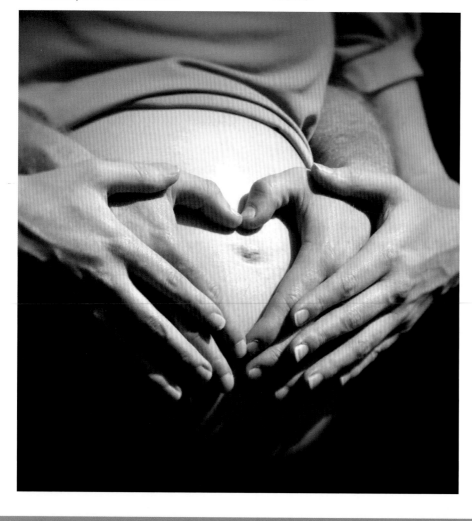
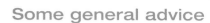

conceiving over the following year.

Therefore, the usual pre-conception advice still applies. For example, women are advised to:

⇨ Take folic acid each day to reduce the chance of a spinal cord problem in a baby.

⇨ Have a blood test to check that they are immune to rubella (German measles). They will be offered immunisation to rubella if they are not immune.

⇨ Eat a healthy diet.

In addition, the following may be relevant to some people:

⇨ Smoking can affect fertility in men and women. It has been estimated that in each menstrual cycle, smokers have about two thirds the chance of conceiving compared to non-smokers. Smoking is also harmful to a developing baby if the mother smokes. Therefore, it is a good time for both partners to stop if you are smokers.

⇨ Alcohol in excess may affect fertility. Also the Department of Health recommends that women trying to become

pregnant do not drink any alcohol. However, the exact amount of alcohol that is safe during pregnancy is not known. This is why the advice is not to drink at all. If you do choose to drink when trying to become pregnant then limit it to one or two units, once or twice a week. (This is the equivalent of one or two glasses of wine, once or twice a week.) You should never binge drink or get drunk. This is because alcohol may harm a developing baby.

⇨ Weight control. You have a reduced chance of conceiving if you are very overweight or underweight. For the best chance of conceiving, you should aim to have your body mass index (BMI) at between 20 and 30. If appropriate, see your practice nurse to measure your BMI and for advice about diet and weight control.

⇨ Some street drugs can affect fertility and are best avoided.

⇨ Heat and sperm production. It is often advised for men who have a low sperm count to wear loose-fitting underpants and trousers and to avoid very hot baths, saunas, etc.

This allows your testes to be slightly cooler than the rest of your body, which is thought to be good for sperm production. It is not clear whether these measures actually do improve sperm count, but they seem to be sensible.

"Older women tend to be less fertile than younger women. The fall off of fertility seems to be greatest once you are past your middle 30s"

What are the main treatments used for infertility?

Fertility treatments can be grouped into three categories:

⇨ Medicines to improve fertility – these are sometimes used alone, but can also be used in addition to assisted conception.

⇨ Surgical treatments – these may be used when a cause of the infertility is found that may be helped by an operation.

⇨ Assisted conception – this includes several techniques such as intrauterine insemination (IUI), in vitro fertilisation (IVF), gamete intrafallopian transfer (GIFT), and intracytoplasmic sperm injection (ICSI).

14 June 2012

⇨ The above information was originally written by Dr Tim Kenny. The current version is authored by Dr Hayley Willacy. The article is reproduced with kind permission from EMIS. Please visit www.patient.co.uk for further information.

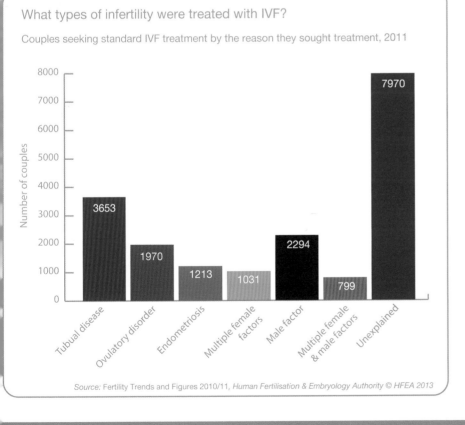

What types of infertility were treated with IVF?

Couples seeking standard IVF treatment by the reason they sought treatment, 2011

Source: Fertility Trends and Figures 2010/11, Human Fertilisation & Embryology Authority © HFEA 2013

© EMIS 2013

Common fertility myths

There are lots of myths and misinformation about infertility and its causes. Here's the low-down on what's true and what's not.

If you have concerns about fertility, the last thing you want is a lot of bad information from friends and family about its causes and effects. There are lots of Old Wives' Tales to do with having babies – but what's true and what's a load of old rubbish?

Myth: if you have fertility treatment, you'll have twins or triplets

It was certainly true in the past that if you had fertility treatment and had several embryos put into your womb, you might have had several babies at the end of it. This used to happen because in many cases, only one or two embryos would become a viable baby. Of course, if all the babies were viable, you could end up with a multiple pregnancy! However, this situation has now changed. The Human Fertilisation and Embryology Association (HFEA) has changed the guidelines on the number of embryos put into a woman's womb to avoid this (as a multiple pregnancy puts a huge strain on the mother) and now, women are often implanted with just one or at most two embryos. This, together with increases in the success rate for IVF pregnancies, means multiple births are now not such a risk.

Myth: conceiving a second baby is easy if you've already had one

If you conceived your first baby quickly and easily with no delays and no problems, you may assume that it will be just as easy a second time. But that's not always the case. If your first pregnancy was after a delay or you had to have fertility treatment, you may already be worried about trying again. Additional factors such as tiredness and stress due to having a child don't help, either and many people put pressure on themselves to conceive at a certain time to fit in with work or to get a certain age gap between the children.

Many women experience what is called 'secondary infertility' where they have problems getting pregnant with a second child. It may not mean that anything is wrong but if you have been trying for a while, or if you are significantly older than when you had your first baby, you might want to ask your doctor to refer you for tests.

Myth: older women need fertility treatment to get pregnant

This is at least based on a little bit of truth as your fertility does decline and if you're over 35, you might find it more difficult to get pregnant than a 25-year-old woman. But many women of that age and older conceive naturally and with no problems.

If you are an older woman and are having problems getting pregnant, ask your doctor if you would be suitable to be referred for fertility treatment.

Myth: infertility is always the woman's fault

Firstly, it is nobody's 'fault'. Fertility problems may be as a result of a physical problem or a previous medical condition but are not something that the person could have wanted or predicted. And secondly, there are as many causes in infertility in men as there are in women, so it is essential that you are both tested at an early stage.

Myth: stress causes infertility

Whilst trying for a baby can be stressful and going month after month with no blue line on the pregnancy test kit makes it worse, fertility problems are physical and need to be diagnosed and treated.

Myth: daily sex will help you get pregnant quickly

Sounds to good to be true? That's because it is! Your eggs are released at a certain time each month – usually 14 – 16 days before your next period – and healthy sperm can remain alive for up to 72 hours. So you have a small window of a few days each month when conception is possible. Of course, if you have irregular periods or your partner has a low sperm count, it may not be so easy to predict when you are both at your most fertile. Above all, make sure you don't put pressure on yourselves.

2 September 2011

⇨ The above information is reprinted with kind permission from Bounty (UK) Ltd. Please visit www.bounty.com for further information.

Protect your fertility

Age is an important factor when it comes to getting pregnant, especially for women, but everyone can help to protect their fertility.

Even if babies are the last thing on your mind at the moment, you can take steps to help maintain your fertility.

Professor William Ledger, Professor of Obstetrics and Gynaecology at the University of Sheffield, explains the basics.

Age and fertility

When it comes to fertility, age matters.

Many people today wait until they're older to have children. But fertility declines over time, and you should consider this if you plan to have children later.

Both women and men are at their most fertile in their early 20s.

In women, fertility declines more quickly with age. This decline becomes rapid after the age of 35. This has a number of causes, but particularly the decline in the quality of the eggs released by the ovaries.

Around one-third of couples in which the woman is over 35 have fertility problems. This rises to two-thirds when the woman is over 40.

Women over 35 are also less likely to become pregnant as a result of fertility treatments, including IVF, and are more likely to have a miscarriage if they do become pregnant.

Men's fertility gradually declines from around the age of 40, but most men are able to father children into their 50s and beyond.

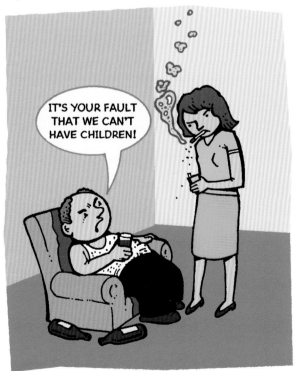

IT'S YOUR FAULT THAT WE CAN'T HAVE CHILDREN!

Good fertility health

Other factors also affect fertility. But, in many cases, you can take action to help protect your fertility.

Avoid STIs

Sexually transmitted infections, such as chlamydia and gonorrhoea, can damage a woman's fallopian tubes, which may make it more difficult to become pregnant. If you think you might have contracted an STI, go to your GP or a sexual health clinic. Find out more about STIs.

Don't smoke

'Women who smoke 20 cigarettes a day experience the menopause on average two years earlier,' says Professor Ledger. Men who smoke risk damaging their sperm. Get advice on stopping smoking.

Be a healthy weight

Being underweight or overweight can lower your chances of conceiving. One cause of infertility is polycystic ovary syndrome (PCOS), which is made worse by being overweight or obese. You can check whether you're a healthy weight with a healthy weight calculator.

Drink sensibly

The government advises against drinking alcohol if you are trying to get pregnant. Women trying to get pregnant can reduce the risk of harming a developing baby by not drinking to excess and drinking no more than one or two units of alcohol once or twice a week.

Men who exceed three to four units a day may damage their sperm.

Keep your testicles cool

A man's testicles should be one or two degrees cooler than the rest of his body. Tight underwear, hot showers and hot baths can all raise the temperature of the testicles.

Avoid radiation and dangerous chemicals

Exposure to radiation and chemicals such as glycol ester, found in some paints, can damage fertility.

Fertility problems

Your GP can do tests to identify possible fertility problems, and can provide advice on the next steps.

4 October 2012

⇨ The above information is reprinted with kind permission from NHS Choices. Please visit www.nhs.uk for further information.

Men have a ticking biological clock too, says study

It's not just women who have a ticking biological clock, according to a study that has found the chances of men fathering children fall with every passing year once they reach middle age.

By Martin Beckford, health correspondent

Analysis of patients at an infertility clinic found that the chances of a man getting his wife pregnant dropped by seven per cent each year between the ages of 41 and 45, reducing even more sharply among older men.

The quality of the husband's sperm was also found to deteriorate with time.

Until now the pressure has been on women to start a family before they turn 40, when the chances of them getting pregnant naturally or artificially start to decline sharply as their reserves of eggs run low and their quality declines.

But experts say that men should not leave it too late either if they want to be sure of having children.

Lead researcher Dr Paula Fettback, of the Huntingdon Reproductive Medicine Centre in Brazil, said: 'Of course it's not the same as for women, but men can't wait for ever. After 45 if they haven't, they have to start thinking about having children.'

In the study, presented this week at the annual conference of the American Society for Reproductive Medicine in Florida, she analysed the outcome of 570 IVF treatments carried out at her clinic between March 2008 and April this year.

To make sure that the age of the woman did not skew the study, only cases where eggs were donated by young healthy women were included.

The results showed that the age of men in the group that did not conceive was 'significantly higher' than among those who were able to have a baby.

Further analysis found that when the husband was 41, the couple had a 60 per cent chance of getting pregnant.

'Our regression analysis also showed that every additional year on a husband's age may reduce the odds of pregnancy in seven per cent.'

By age 45 the chances were said to be down to 35 per cent, and dropped more sharply thereafter.

In addition, the morphology or shape of the sperm was better in the pregnant group.

Dr Fettback said: 'The contribution of female age on human reproduction is well known however the contribution of male age is not well understood.

'As a growing number of men are choosing to father children at older ages, comprehending the impact of male age and sperm quality has become incredibly important in public health.'

Separate research in mice, presented at the same meeting, showed that only a 35 per cent of those who were 'middle-aged' impregnated females, down from three-quarters among younger males. Many of the pregnancies in older mice also led to miscarriage.

Charles Kingsland, a consultant gynaecologist at Liverpool Women's Hospital who is a leading member of the British Fertility Society, said the Brazilian study should be treated with caution as it was small and carried out retrospectively.

He added that men produce fresh sperm every day, compared with women who are born with a lifetime supply of eggs, but their quality could be damaged by unhealthy diet, smoking or obesity.

'There are lots of advantages to being a younger father, first and foremost you have more energy, but being an older father does confer certain advantages such as stability, wisdom and maybe a bit more financial security.'

20 October 2011

⇨ The above information is reprinted with kind permission from *The Telegraph*. Please visit www.telegraph.co.uk for further information.

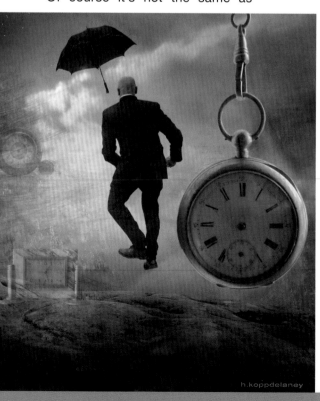

h.koppdelaney

Fertility treatment options

In vitro fertilisation (IVF)

What is it?

In vitro fertilisation (IVF) literally means 'fertilisation in glass' giving us the familiar term 'test tube baby'.

During the IVF process, eggs are removed from the ovaries and fertilised with sperm in the laboratory. The fertilised egg (embryo) is later placed in the woman's womb.

The risks

Drug reaction

A mild reaction to fertility drugs may involve hot flushes, feeling down or irritable, headaches and restlessness.

Ovarian hyper-stimulation syndrome (OHSS)

OHSS can be a dangerous over-reaction to fertility drugs used to stimulate egg production. It can cause symptoms such as a swollen stomach, stomach pains, nausea and vomiting.

Miscarriage

Although the risk of a miscarriage after IVF is no higher than after a natural conception, nor is the risk lower. To check that the pregnancy is not likely to miscarry an ultrasound scan is usually done about two weeks after the positive pregnancy test.

Ectopic pregnancy

When an embryo develops in your fallopian tube rather than your womb, the pregnancy is said to be ectopic. Hormone tests and scans are used to detect ectopic pregnancies

Intra-cytoplasmic sperm injection (ICSI)

What is it?

Intra-cytoplasmic sperm injection (ICSI) involves injecting a single sperm directly into an egg in order to fertilise it. The fertilised egg (embryo) is then transferred to the woman's womb.

The major development of ICSI means that as long as some sperm can be obtained (even in very low numbers), fertilisation is possible.

The risks

Because ICSI is a fairly new treatment (it was introduced in 1992), it is not yet known whether there is any risk that injecting the sperm into an egg could damage it, with possible long-term consequences for the child.

The risks that have so far been associated with ICSI are:

⇨ Certain genetic and developmental defects in a very small number of children born using this treatment. However, problems that have been linked with ICSI may have been caused by the underlying infertility, rather than the technique itself.

⇨ The possibility that a boy conceived as a result of ICSI may inherit his father's infertility. It is too early to know if this is the case, as the oldest boys born from ICSI are still in their early teens.

⇨ An increased risk of miscarriage because the technique uses sperm that would not otherwise have been able to fertilise an egg.

⇨ A low sperm count caused by genetic problems could be passed on to a male child, so you may want to undergo genetic tests before going ahead with ICSI. Infertile men with low sperm count or no sperm in their ejaculate may be tested for cystic fibrosis genes and for chromosome abnormalities. You may want to discuss the full implications of taking these tests with your clinician or the clinic's counsellor before going ahead.

Intrauterine insemination (IUI)

What is it?

Intrauterine insemination (IUI) involves a laboratory procedure to separate fast-moving-sperm from more sluggish or non-moving sperm.

The fast moving sperm are then placed into the woman's womb close to the time of ovulation when the egg is released from the ovary in the middle of the monthly cycle.

The risks

IUI itself is normally quite straightforward – it is usually fairly painless, although you may experience mild cramps similar to period pains.

However, the risks associated with the fertility drugs that are often used with this treatment can include reactions to the drugs and certain pregnancy problems.

With stimulated IUI, this also run the risk of multiple pregnancy.

The use of ultrasound scanning before ovulation means that if there are more than two mature egg follicles present, the cycle can be abandoned.

Donor insemination (DI)

What is it?

Donor insemination (DI) uses sperm from a donor to help the woman become pregnant.

Sperm donors are screened for sexually transmitted diseases and some genetic disorders. In DI, sperm from the donor is placed into the neck of the womb (cervix) at the time when the woman ovulates.

The risks

The risks associated with DI treatment depend on how it is used:

⇨ where DI is combined with the use of fertility drugs, the risk of multiple births is increased. After conception, the risks are the same as those for normal pregnancies

⇨ if you are using donor sperm with IVF, the same risks apply

⇨ using sperm from sources other than a registered donor is not only dangerous but illegal. Only sperm from registered donors should be used for DI, as this ensures the donor will have been thoroughly screened for many sexually transmitted and some hereditary diseases and the sperm will have been quarantined for six months (to check that the sample is not infected with diseases such as HIV and hepatitis B and C) before use.

Genetic testing

What is it?

Pre-implantation genetic testing involves carrying out tests on embryos created through IVF or ICSI to detect certain inherited conditions or abnormalities.

This helps to ensure that only unaffected embryos are selected before they are transferred to the womb.

Conventional pre-natal tests for genetic diseases cannot be carried out until the 12th week of pregnancy.

Testing embryos before they are implanted could help couples avoid having to make the difficult decision whether to have an abortion if either is the carrier of a genetic condition and the embryo is affected.

The risks

With pre-implantation genetic diagnosis (PGD), there is also the possibility that:

⇨ some embryos may be damaged by the process of cell removal

⇨ testing may not be 100% reliable or conclusive.

Problems unique to pre-implantation genetic screening (PGS) treatment include:

⇨ some embryos may be damaged by the process of cell removal

⇨ possibility that no embryos are suitable for transfer to the womb after PGS.

Gamete intra-fallopian transfer (GIFT)

What is it?

With gamete intra-fallopian transfer (GIFT), the preparation and monitoring of the growth of eggs is identical to IVF.

Instead of the eggs being fertilised 'in vitro' in the laboratory, the healthiest eggs and sperm are placed together in the woman's fallopian tubes. Fertilisation therefore takes place in the body, as it would if conception had occurred naturally.

The risks

As much of the treatment is similar to in vitro fertilisation IVF, the risks with gamete intra-fallopian transfer (GIFT) are also similar, including the possibility of reactions to drugs and multiple births.

GIFT, also has the added risks that are a part of any procedure that involves the use of a general anaesthetic and surgery.

There are also the particular risks of laparoscopy ('keyhole surgery' – minimal invasive surgery without having to make large incisions – which allows a surgeon to view organs in the abdomen through the abdomen wall using a fibre-optic instrument). Although it is a rare complication, trauma to structures in the abdomen can occur during the insertion process of the laparoscope.

In vitro maturation (IVM)

What is it?

With in vitro maturation (IVM) eggs are removed from the ovaries and are collected when they are still immature. They are then matured in the laboratory before being fertilised.

The difference between IVM and conventional IVF is that the eggs are immature when they are collected. This means that the woman does not need to take as many drugs before the eggs can be collected as she might if using conventional IVF, when mature eggs are collected.

The risks

As IVM is a new technique, there is not enough evidence to be absolutely certain of its safety as the number of children born is very few – about 400 worldwide – and those that have been born are still very young.

The known risks of IVM are:

⇨ fewer eggs are collected than in conventional IVF

⇨ the usual risks involved in having a general anaesthetic.

A clinic would suggest IVM because they consider that patient's susceptibility to ovarian hyper-stimulation syndrome (OHSS) is higher than average.

Reproductive immunology

What is it?

Reproductive immunology is a service offered by a few fertility clinics in the UK. It includes a range of tests and treatment to do with the patient's immune system in pregnancy.

There is much debate about the role of the immune system in promoting or preventing a healthy pregnancy. This information outlines the latest findings and views of experts on the topic so far (to March 2010). It does not reflect studies and views published after it was written.

The risks

These tests and treatments are very new. To date (March 2010), there is little scientific proof that these treatments are effective in improving the chance of having a baby. The little evidence currently available is strongly questioned by other clinicians and experts.

Fertility drugs

What are they?

If a female isn't ovulating properly (producing and releasing an egg each month), fertility drugs – which trigger egg production in much the same way as your body's own hormones – can help. This is known as ovulation induction.

It is possible to get pregnant using fertility drugs alone, or they may be offered alongside other treatments such as IUI and IVF. If they are not used as part of treatment at a licensed fertility clinic, their use is not regulated by the HFEA.

Drugs are not as important in the treatment of male infertility as they are in the treatment of women. However, they may occasionally be prescribed in certain situations, which may include:

⇨ antibiotics to treat infection or inflammation

⇨ vitamins C and E to improve sperm movement, although there is no convincing evidence that this improves the chance of pregnancy

⇨ gonadotrophin injections or pump administration for certain rare conditions in which no sperm is produced

⇨ drugs that close the bladder neck when sperm are being ejaculated into the bladder instead of the penis (retrograde ejaculation).

The risks

Apart from the risks of the side-effects of common fertility drugs, such as mood swings, nausea, stomach pains, etc., taking fertility drugs increases the chance of a multiple pregnancy and birth.

14 April 2007–9 January 2013

⇨ The above information is reprinted with kind permission from the Human Fertilisation & Embryology Authority (HFEA). Please visit www.hfea.gov.uk for further information.

© HFEA 2013

In vitro fertilisation

In vitro fertilisation (IVF) is one of several techniques available to help couples with fertility problems to have a baby.

How IVF is performed

The IVF technique was developed in the 1970s. It may differ slightly from clinic to clinic but a typical treatment is as follows.

For women

Step one: suppressing the natural monthly cycle

You are given a drug that will suppress your natural menstrual cycle. This is given either as a daily injection (which you'll be taught to give yourself) or as a nasal spray. You continue this for about two weeks.

Step two: boosting the egg supply

Once your natural cycle is suppressed, you take a fertility hormone called FSH (follicle stimulating hormone). These fertility hormones are known as gonadotrophins. This is another daily injection that you give yourself, usually for about 12 days, but it can vary depending on your response.

FSH increases the number of eggs your ovaries produce. This means that more eggs can be collected and fertilised. With more fertilised eggs, the clinic has a greater choice of embryos to use in your treatment.

Step three: checking on progress

The clinic will keep an eye on you throughout the drug treatment. You will have vaginal ultrasound scans to monitor your ovaries and, in some cases, blood tests. About 34–36 hours before your eggs are due to be collected, you'll have a final hormone injection that helps your eggs to mature.

Step four: collecting the eggs

For the egg collection, you'll be sedated and your eggs will be collected under ultrasound guidance. This involves a needle being inserted through the vagina and into each ovary. The eggs are then collected through the needle.

Some women experience cramps or a small amount of vaginal bleeding after the procedure.

Step five: fertilising the eggs

The eggs that have been collected are mixed with your partner's or the donor's sperm in the laboratory. After 16–20 hours they're checked to see if any have been fertilised.

If the sperm are few or weak, each egg may need to be injected individually with a single sperm. This is called intra-cytoplasmic sperm injection or ICSI (see below). In 2008, over 40% of all IVF procedures used the ICSI technique.

The cells that have been fertilised (embryos) continue to grow in the laboratory for one to five days before being transferred into the womb. The best one or two embryos will be chosen for transfer.

After egg collection, you will be given medicines, either progesterone or hCG (chorionic gonadotrophin), to help prepare the lining of the womb to receive the embryo. This is given either as a pessary (which is placed inside the vagina) or an injection.

Step six: embryo transfer

The number of embryos to be replaced should have been discussed before treatment starts.

Women under 37 in their first IVF cycle should only have a single embryo transfer. In their second IVF cycle they should have a single embryo transfer if one or more top-quality embryos are available. Doctors should only consider using two embryos if no top-quality embryos are available. In the third IVF cycle, no more than two embryos should be transferred.

Women aged 37–39 years in the first and second full IVF cycles should also have single embryo transfer if there are one or more top-quality embryos, and double embryo transfer should only be considered if there are no top-quality embryos.

In the third cycle, no more than two embryos should be transferred.

For women aged 40-42 years, double embryo transfer can be considered.

All multiple embryo replacements carry the risk of a multiple pregnancy and birth. Multiple pregnancies are associated with a significantly increased risk of premature labour, resulting in a three- to five-fold increased risk of blindness, deafness and cerebral palsy.

If any embryos are left over, and they're suitable, they may be frozen for future IVF attempts (see HFEA: freezing and storing embryos).

Some clinics may also offer a process called blastocyst transfer. This is where the fertilised eggs are left to mature for five to six days before being transferred.

For men

Around the time your partner's eggs are collected, you'll be asked to produce a fresh sample of sperm. The sperm are washed and spun at a high speed, so the healthiest and most active sperm can be selected.

If you're using donated sperm, it is removed from frozen storage, thawed and prepared in the same way.

Information on other techniques

There are many alternative methods to help a couple conceive. For more information, see the HFEA factsheets on:

⇨ natural cycle IVF – IVF without fertility drugs and hormones to boost the supply of eggs

⇨ intra-cytoplasmic sperm injection (ICSI) – injecting a single sperm directly into an egg to fertilise it

⇨ intrauterine insemination (IUI) – separating fast-moving sperm from more sluggish or non-moving sperm

⇨ gamete intra-fallopian transfer (GIFT) – placing the healthiest eggs and sperm together in the woman's fallopian tubes so that fertilisation takes place in the body

⇨ in vitro maturation (IVM) – maturing the eggs in the laboratory before fertilising them

Who can have IVF?

In 2013, the National Institute for Health and Clinical Excellence (NICE) published new guidelines about who should have access to IVF treatment on the NHS in England and Wales.

Women under 40

According to the guidelines, women under 40 years should be offered three cycles of IVF treatment on the NHS if:

⇨ you have been trying to get pregnant through regular unprotected intercourse for two years, or

⇨ you have not been able to get pregnant after 12 cycles of artificial insemination

However, if tests show that IVF is the only treatment likely to help you get pregnant, you should be referred for IVF straight away.

If you turn 40 during treatment, the current cycle will be completed, but further cycles should not be offered.

Women aged 40 to 42

The guidelines also say that women aged between 40 and 42 should be offered one cycle of IVF on the NHS if all of the following four criteria are met:

⇨ you have been trying to get pregnant through regular unprotected intercourse for a total of two years, or you have not been able to get pregnant after 12 cycles of artificial insemination

⇨ you have never had IVF treatment before

⇨ you show no evidence of low ovarian reserve (this is when eggs in the ovary are impaired or low in number)

⇨ you have been informed of the additional implications of IVF and pregnancy at this age.

Again, if tests show that IVF is the only treatment likely to help you get pregnant, you should be referred for IVF straight away.

Success rate

The success rate of IVF depends on the age of the woman undergoing treatment as well as the cause of the infertility (if it's known). Younger women are more likely to have healthier eggs, which increases the chances of success.

IVF isn't usually recommended for women above the age of 42 because the chances of a successful pregnancy are thought to be too low.

In 2010, the percentage IVF treatments that resulted in a live birth (the success rate) was:

⇨ 32.2% for women under 35

⇨ 27.7% for women aged 35–37

⇨ 20.8% for women aged 38–39

⇨ 13.6% for women aged 40–42

⇨ 5% for women aged 43–44

⇨ 1.9% for women aged over 44

Funding and payment

NHS trusts across England and Wales are working to provide the same levels of service. However, the provision of IVF treatment varies across the country and it often depends on local trust policies. Priority is often given to couples who don't already have children.

If you're not eligible for NHS funding or you decide to pay for IVF, you can approach a private fertility clinic directly. On average, one cycle of IVF costs about £5,000. However, this varies from clinic to clinic and there may be additional costs for medicines, consultations and tests.

Some clinics may offer a 'package' of treatment. During your discussions with the clinic, make sure you find out exactly what's included in the price. You may also be able to reduce the cost of IVF by donating some of your eggs for others to use.

⇨ The above information is reprinted with kind permission from NHS Choices. Please visit www.nhs.uk for further information.

© NHS Choices 2013

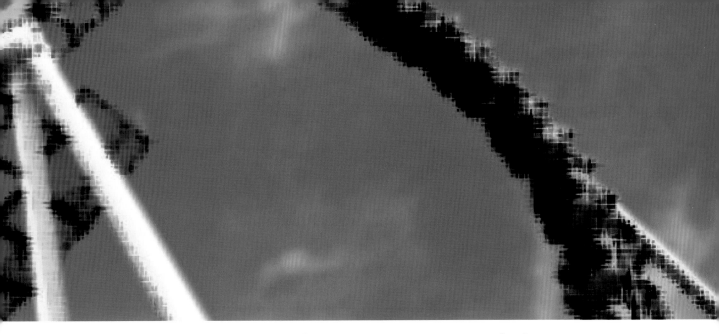

IVF treatment – roller coaster ride

Listed in Women's Health, originally published in Issue 169 – April 2010.

By Kate Arnold

Having been sterilised in January 1998, I'd been told that my more likely chance of having a baby, eight years later, would be IVF.

As I already had children from a previous relationship, I was told that there would be no financial assistance from the NHS and that I would have to attend a private hospital.

October 2006 was our first appointment with the Consultant Paediatrician (who was the same man that I had seen at my local hospital), where we discussed the options of which type of IVF we would need.

And so the regime started. Tablets every day for three months to prepare my body for possible pregnancy, followed by injections every day in my leg.

The injections started off well. No problem in doing them myself, until one day, I just froze and wasn't able to do any more. I felt like a failure! Why was I suddenly being so silly? I had the syringe ready. I had a clean leg. What was the problem? I just couldn't do it and I felt stupid.

Later that day, I had an appointment at the hospital and explained what had happened and how upset I'd got myself over it. They were fantastic and did the injections for me when my husband couldn't.

Once I'd had the all the injections and my body was ready for the eggs to be collected, I went into hospital to have the eggs removed from me.

The doctors kept my eggs in their incubators, mixed it with my husband's sperm and waited! They wait to see which eggs are the best and have the best chance of survival.

Back I go to hospital to have the eggs re-implanted in me. I'd been told that I had 17 taken from me and they were going to give me back three. They said that those three looked really good and healthy. I did wonder how they could possibly look healthy???

IVF is a constant waiting game.

Once the eggs were back in, I had to wait two weeks before I could do a pregnancy test. Having already gone through pregnancy before, good healthy pregnancies, I honestly felt that everything would be just fine. I felt that there was no reason whatsoever that it wouldn't work.

I did my pregnancy test. POSITIVE! I knew it would be OK. They booked me for a scan for two weeks later. I was so pleased. I went for the scan at the hospital two weeks later alone, as I thought that as it would be so tiny, there would be nothing for my husband to see or do.

As I sat in the waiting room, just before they called me in, I knew. I knew that something was wrong. I have no idea how I knew that. One of the strangest things ever for me was that feeling. I went in, got changed and then she started the scanning, and told me what I had already just figured out. The baby that was meant to be growing steadily had no heart beat. I suddenly felt numb. She apologised to me. Not her fault. I got dressed and was then told that I would need to come back again in two more weeks just to be doubly sure that it had indeed died and then we could move on to the next procedure.

My husband and I returned two weeks later; they had been right the first time and there was no heart beat. I cried. A lot. A few weeks later, I had to go into hospital again and have it removed.

I swore I wouldn't go through it again. What a painful experience it was. I'd told my husband, who didn't have any children, that I would never do it again.

A year later, a new house, new challenges, I changed my mind. I told my husband and myself that one last go and that would be it. I really would not do it a third time.

So, it started all over again. This time though I had to go on the pill for three months in preparation. Then I had to have more drugs. The toll this was taking on my moods was no one's business. I'm not the most placid of people at the best of times, but these drugs made me so moody.

The injections started again and I didn't do any of them myself. After the last time, I didn't even try them. My husband would do them daily before work, and when he was away, my eldest daughter did them. I think she enjoyed it!

This time, I was prepared for the worst. I knew the risks and understood that it might not work.

11 February 2008. Egg implantation day.

All went well and according to plan. They told me at the hospital what to do for the next few days. No lifting, take painkillers and rest.

Two weeks went by and I did my pregnancy test again. POSITIVE. This time I didn't think that everything would be OK and knew that it could all go horribly wrong. We had to wait three weeks before the scan. I just needed to know

what, if anything, was happening inside me. I'd told my husband that he had to come to the scan with me, otherwise I wasn't going. He came.

The scan started as normal, searching round my insides to find what it is they need to find. Yes, she says, we have a heart beat. I was so pleased. That was one hurdle over. She keeps turning the probe and then she says, we have a second heart beat. Oh my God. I just squeezed my husband's hand and looked at him, not sure whether to laugh or cry. Then she says that she had to get a colleague. They return and keep probing, and we're starting to get worried. Then she says, we have a third heart beat. Then a little tear fell from my eye. My husband and I just looked at each other, unsure what to say. She showed us the monitor and sure enough, three little people with heart beats.

By 14 weeks, I was in maternity clothes as I was gaining so much weight. I found that odd, as I didn't have much of an appetite. I couldn't lie down flat because my blood pressure would get too low, and I found it very difficult to sleep at night.

During one of my many scans, I was told that there was a lot of fluid

round my belly which would need to be kept an eye on, and that was that. At the ante-natal appointment later on, the Consultant told me that they suspected that the identical twins inside me had Twin to Twin Transfusion Syndrome and that I would need to go to London to see Professor Nickolaides, who is one of the world's best experts with this particular syndrome, and he would decide what to do.

When we saw him a few days later we were told that the receiving twin was too big, and also that if it survived, would have a heart condition, and that the donor twin wasn't getting enough blood or oxygen. The worst bit was that if I didn't have laser surgery then and there, the chances of survival were next to nothing; with the surgery chances of all three babies surviving was only 3%.

We took the chance. They split the placenta of the twin babies to give them both a fighting chance. They also drained two litres of fluid from my belly. It meant that I could sleep again and eat properly.

It didn't work. Two days later, triplet one died. I was 19 weeks along.

I wasn't able to work after that as I was at high risk of miscarriage.

At 25 weeks and six days, I went into labour.

At 26 weeks exactly, Amelia and Chloe came into this world. 1 lb 14 oz and 1 lb 8 oz.

What a fight and struggle they both had.

My beautiful Chloe didn't last past ten weeks. She had so many different problems she couldn't fight anymore.

Amelia is 18 months old and doing just fine. Would I do IVF again?

NEVER!

⇨ The above information is reprinted with kind permission from Positive Health Online. Please visit www.positivehealth. com for further information.

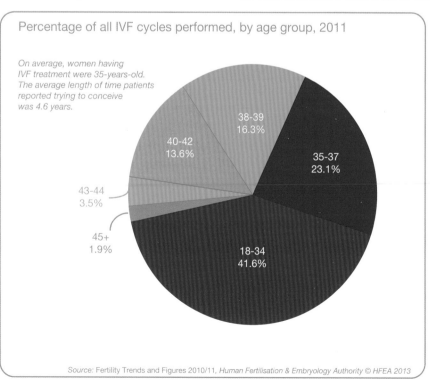

Percentage of all IVF cycles performed, by age group, 2011

On average, women having IVF treatment were 35-years-old. The average length of time patients reported trying to conceive was 4.6 years.

38-39
16.3%

40-42
13.6%

35-37
23.1%

43-44
3.5%

45+
1.9%

18-34
41.6%

Source: Fertility Trends and Figures 2010/11, Human Fertilisation & Embryology Authority © HFEA 2013

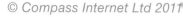

Five million IVF babies born to date, study says

By Suzanne Elvidge

Back in July 1978, Leslie Brown became the proud mother of her first child, Louise. The birth of a single baby girl may not sound like groundbreaking news, but Louise was the first baby created by IVF. A study now estimates that she has been joined by another five million people worldwide born thanks to assisted reproductive technologies (ART).

This figure was presented at the 28th annual meeting of the European Society of Human Reproduction and Embryology (ESHRE) in Istanbul, Turkey, and includes babies born after IVF and ICSI. In the latter technique, the sperm is injected directly into the egg as a step of IVF.

Dr Allan Pacey, chairman of the British Fertility Society, told BBC News: 'I think it's significant that we've got to five million. It's far more socially acceptable than it has been over the last ten or 20 years.'

Talking to the *Daily Telegraph*, he added: 'I think it's more than just older women relying on IVF. I think it's more about accessibility, social acceptability, funding issues and, to an extent, that IVF is part of the mainstream now.'

The International Committee for Monitoring ART (ICMART) calculated the numbers by using reported figures from 1978 to 2008, and then estimating figures for 2009 to 2012. ICMART data suggest that around 1.5 million ART cycles are now performed globally each year, leading to around 350,000 babies, and the numbers are rising.

But such data does show how many failures there still are in IVF treatment. Stuart Lavery, a consultant gynaecologist and director of IVF at Hammersmith Hospital, told BBC News that advances in IVF could lead people to 'view IVF as an insurance policy that they can access at any stage. Unfortunately the facts still suggest that IVF success rates in women as they get older are not fantastic'.

The ICMART data further illustrates how demand for IVF continues to grow. In Europe 532,260 IVF treatment cycles were performed in 2008, increasing to 537,287 in 2009.

Leslie Brown, Louise Brown's mother, died last month. She had a second daughter through IVF, Natalie (the 40th IVF baby), as well as a stepdaughter and five grandchildren. Natalie was the first person conceived via IVF to have a child herself (conceived naturally) and Louise also has a naturally-conceived child.

Dr Simon Fishel, managing director of CARE Fertility, UK, and a member of the Edwards and Steptoe group in Cambridge responsible for the birth of Louise Brown said: 'I remember well the time of Louise's birth, and also transferring the embryo that became her sister – both of whom are now mums in their own right. The five million milestone not only justifies all the legal and moral battles, the ethical debates and hard-fought social approval, it is also a testament to the great scientists and doctors who have worked so hard to improve the treatment of patients, and to the patients themselves who have put their faith in us.'

Sources & references

⇨ Five million IVF babies since 1978 *Daily Telegraph*, 2 July 2012

⇨ Five millionth 'test tube baby' BBC News, 2 July 2012

⇨ Successful IVF births reach five million Independent, 2 July 2012

⇨ The world's number of IVF and ICSI babies has now reached a calculated total of five million European Society of Human Reproduction and Embryology (ESHRE), 2 July 2012

02 July 2012

⇨ The above information is reprinted with kind permission from BioNews. Please visit www.bionews.org.uk for further information.

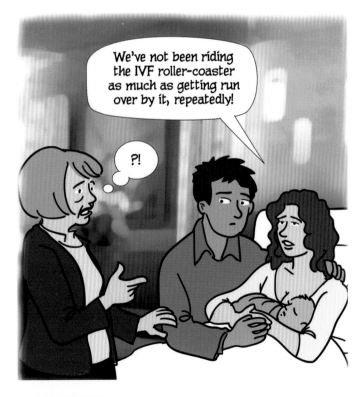

We've not been riding the IVF roller-coaster as much as getting run over by it, repeatedly!

?!

Adoption

Details of the adoption process.

By Dr Marcus

What is involved in the adoption of a child?

Adoption is providing a family for a child who can not be brought up by his or her biological parents. Adoption is a legal process that will make the adopted parents fully responsible of the adopted child by law. Legal adoption began in England and Wales in 1962 and in Scotland in 1930, with the first adoption acts. Once an adoption order has been granted, it can not be reversed except in extremely rare circumstances. In the United States, approximately 120,000 children are adopted annually with nearly 50% of the children adopted by relatives.

Over the past decade, the number of babies available for adoption has declined dramatically. The legal and social requirements are numerous whether the adopted child is within the UK or overseas. Couples seeking adoptions have to come to terms with their infertility and may have a period of grief before seeing adoption as a positive alternative. Although most families seek adoption because of infertility, some seek adoption because they desire more children.

Adoption requires both partners to be heavily involved, committed and positive. For those women who feel deeply that a part of their life has escaped them as they did not enjoy the months of pregnancy and did not go through the pain of labour and the pleasure of childbirth, for them adoption may not be a good option.

Adopted parents should be prepared to accept emotional reactions as the arrival of the adopted child may reawaken feelings of their grief over their infertility, emotions to which they had worked very hard in the past years to overcome. It may also be a reminder of their failure and inability to bear their own children. The adopted parents may feel guilty about their own emotions, when they are trying to establish a loving relationship with their adopted child. As that new loving relationship starts to develop and intensify, the grief will gradually disappear.

All children who are adopted should know that they are adopted. Discovery or disclosure of adoption when the child is older can lead to mistrust and anger, etc. The process of telling the child that he or she was adopted should take place gradually.

There are many ways to adopt each adoption experience is different, parents adopt through public or private agencies that exist for the purpose of finding homes for children in need. Adoption agencies are able to provide counselling, support services and follow up. Private adoptions have more liberal polices and shorter waiting lists.

Adoption in the United Kingdom

The law in the UK requires the adopted parents to be over 21 years old. There is no upper age limit. Potential parents will be expected to show that they can offer the child the care he or she may need. Most agencies want to place healthy babies with couples who have been married for at least three years and have proven they are unable to have children themselves. Some agencies give an upper age limits between 35–40 for adoption of 0–5 years. Older couples are encouraged to adopt older children. Single people are permitted to adopt by UK law and gay and lesbian couples may be approved as adopters.

What is needed to adopt a child in the United Kingdom?

The following is the protocol that may be followed by infertile couples seeking adoption in the UK.

Who can apply to adopt?

The following are eligible to apply to adopt:

⇨ single people (irrespective of their sexual orientation)

⇨ a partner of a parent of the child to be adopted

⇨ married couples

⇨ civil partners

⇨ unmarried couples (same sex and different sex) living as partners in a stable family relationship.

A child's eligibility for adoption

⇨ The child was under the age of 18 when the adoption application was made

⇨ The child is not or has never been married or in a civil partnership

⇨ Both birth parents have given their consent to the adoption

⇨ The birth parent or guardian cannot be found or is incapable of giving consent

⇨ The child's welfare would be at risk if the adoption order was delayed.

The first step a couple seeking adoption must take is to apply to an adoption agency. Each adoption agency has its own requirements for acceptance, so if your are turned down at one agency another agency may accept your application.

The couple are then assessed and prepared for adoption. All prospective parents seeking adoption will undergo an adoption assessment process by the adoption agency. This involves in-depth interviews with the adoption agency. It is a lengthy process and may take up to six months. There is no such thing as the ideal adoptive family. Most agencies are interested in what the prospective parents have to offer a child who needs adoption. Both partners are expected to be in reasonably good physical and mental health. Certification from a family doctor is usually required to show that they have no serious diseases. They may have to undergo a medical examination. Social background is also taken into account, to make sure that the adopted parents have a stable partnership and are able to care for the child materially. Furthermore, a police check may be required.

Finally, a couple must be approved for adoption. Once approved, the agency will try to match the couple with a child. Agencies will always try to match the racial and cultural background of the child, in addition to the child's religion and language, with that of the adoptive parents if possible.

All children and babies should have a complete medical evaluation including growth and development in addition to assessment of immunisation prior to placement for adoption.

Overseas adoption

When local resources have been explored and a scarcity of available children requires a long wait, overseas adoption may be considered. Adopting a child from overseas is neither an easy option nor a quicker route for adoption and involves a lot of patience, careful planning and often a long and tedious legal process. Adoption procedures differ from country to country. The adoption procedure can be very complicated and will vary from case to case. Consultation with a lawyer is advisable to obtain information on the adoption laws, immigration and naturalisation.

In the UK, current information on adoption procedures can be obtained from the Home Office and the Embassy in London for the country that the couple are hoping to adopt from. The adopting parents should ensure from the start that the child is available to be legally adopted. To make this enquiry, adopting parents are advised to go to the social welfare department of the country they wish to adopt from.

> ## "Over the past decade, the number of babies available for adoption has declined dramatically"

The total cost of overseas adoption is between £6,000 to £10,000 in the UK and between $15,000 and $35,000. The costs covers the fees for adoption agency, travel expenses and possibly fees to the authorities in the child country of origin.

12 December 2011

⇨ The above information is reprinted with kind permission from IVF-infertility.com. Please visit www.ivf-infertility.com for further information.

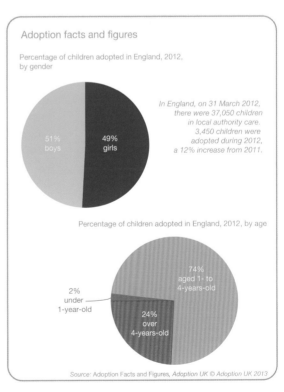

Adoption facts and figures

Percentage of children adopted in England, 2012, by gender

51% boys

49% girls

In England, on 31 March 2012, there were 37,050 children in local authority care. 3,450 children were adopted during 2012, a 12% increase from 2011.

Percentage of children adopted in England, 2012, by age

74% aged 1- to 4-years-old

2% under 1-year-old

24% over 4-years-old

Source: Adoption Facts and Figures, Adoption UK © Adoption UK 2013

Adoption UK's view on some key issues

Here are Adoption UK's positions on several key issues in the adoption field.

Transracial adoption

It is often preferable for the heritage of children and their adopters to be closely matched. However, it is more important that children are placed on timescales that meet their needs (so as avoid further harm or damage via delay), rather than on adult timescales that may be excessively concerned about finding the ideal racial/ethnic match.

Where it is not possible to find a good racial/ethnic match, then adoptive parents will need good quality support services to ensure that their children's heritage is fully reflected as part of the development of their future identity.

Consideration should be given as to whether the child will be part of a community in which at least some people reflect their heritage; how the local community will help the child develop his other identity; what the child will need to know about his or her heritage and what contact will be available with the birth family.

Adoption pay and leave

Current law lays down minimum entitlements to adoption leave and pay but these are less than those for maternity leave and pay. Adoptive parents are discriminated against in three key respects:

⇨ the length of service requirement to be entitled to adoptive leave;

⇨ the rate of pay during the first six weeks of leave; and

⇨ that self-employed adopters have no access to adoption pay while on adoption leave.

Adoption UK is calling for legislation to be amended to give parity between maternity and adoption pay and leave ending the discrimination of those caring for some of the country's most traumatised children.

Social networking/ contact

Increasingly, the security, confidentiality and stability of adoptive families who have adopted children are being undermined by birth families' use of the Internet. Many families who have had their children removed and adopted use the Internet, and sites such as Facebook, as a vehicle to trace the children.

Adopted children can be drawn into Internet communication with their birth families, often inappropriately and dangerously, without protection, support or filters on the veracity of the information they are receiving; and without a full understanding of the implications of re-opening direct contact at a crucial stage of the development of their own identity.

Adoption UK receives countless accounts of the harm and damage caused to adoptive families via this unregulated contact, including potential and actual disruptions and family breakdown.

Reforms of the current recruitment and assessment process

Many prospective adopters are turned away without a proper assessment of their potential as adoptive parents. This can be due to the way that local authorities prioritise their recruitment which is often subject to value judgements on what constitutes a 'good family' – typically a couple with a degree of affluence. Adoption UK has found that out of those prospective adopters who do make it through the application process, too many are subjected to long wait times and bad practice.

Adoption UK is calling for the recruitment of adopters to be a national priority that is implemented nationally rather than locally. Adoption should be promoted positively, and adoptions fully properly and adequately supported.

Contact (general)

The very nature of modern-day adoption means the issue of contact between adopted children and their birth families is extremely complex. Today, the majority of children adopted from the UK care system have been removed from their birth families due to abuse and neglect. The need for practical and emotional support in this area is vital. Research has shown that contact between adopted children and their birth family can be beneficial but it is also recognised that any form of contact needs careful planning and support.

For children who have been removed from their birth families, maintaining some form of contact with them can have major benefits, helping them to develop a healthy sense of identity, understand where they came from and come to terms with their pasts. Contact can be with birth parents, grandparents, brothers and sisters or other members of the family. When a child is adopted, the agency and the adopters agree a contact plan, designed specifically for the child, outlining who they have contact with, how often and in what form.

It should also be noted that contact may not always beneficial to the child; it may, in fact, re-traumatise the child.

Adoption support

Adoption UK believes that the current provision of support services to adopted children and their families is inadequate. Adoptive parents take on some of society's most vulnerable children. They need continuing training and support on child development and how this is affected by the trauma of abuse and neglect, attachment issues and how to be therapeutic parents to abused and neglected children. They also need joined-up, adoption-aware services across not just the social care sector, but also in educational and mental health.

Adoption UK welcomed the publication of the Government's Adoption Action Plan in March 2012 and its focus on improving the adoption system for children in care and their future adoptive families. However, we feel the Action Plan could be strengthened in relation to the development of adoption support services as the aim of recruiting more adopters and placing more children for adoption will not be realised unless support is put in place to help ensure the success of adoptive placements.

Education – why reforms are needed

Adopted children can have periods of distress and difficulty at different stages of their school career due to early trauma they may have experienced.

Currently, adopted children do not receive the same type of entitlements or support as 'looked after' children within schools, e.g. in relation to access to educational support – even though adopted children come from the same population as fostered children. The School Admissions Code was changed in England in December 2011 to give children adopted from the care system the same priority in the school admissions as looked after children.

Adoption UK is campaigning for the same legislation change in Northern Ireland, Scotland and Wales. In addition, adopted children should have the same status as looked after children in relation to their educational need, including entitlements to additional support, across the UK. Adoption UK also believes that educational professionals should be trained in the issues of trauma and attachment.

Overseas adoption

Intercountry adoption is a complex area of law, governed by international conventions and domestic and international law. Someone from the UK who is interested in adopting from overseas has to be prepared, assessed and approved as an adopter in this country, as well as meeting the adoption law requirements of the country from which they want to adopt.

People choose to adopt from overseas for many reasons. They may have a link or previous involvement with, or interest in, a particular country, such as being born there, or lived or worked there, or have family from there, and so on. For some, there may also be the belief that adopting from overseas may be easier, that they will be able to avoid being placed with older, more traumatised children from the UK care system, and/or that they will have more chance of being able to adopt a baby – which is often the starting point for many people when they first think about adoption, as many adopters come from a background of infertility. It is true that overseas adopters will have a better chance of adopting a baby by going overseas, but this does not mean that their adoption will necessarily be easier.

Intercountry adoption is an involved and costly process. Furthermore, children adopted from overseas will share many of the issues of children placed domestically. Both will have had to deal with the traumatising effect of separation from their birth parents, and any associated trauma they may have experienced, which could be due to early abuse/neglect, further changes of carers, all of which will be down to individual circumstances. For overseas adopted children, there may also be questions around the harm caused by being institutionalised in a care home or orphanage.

More fundamentally, however, children adopted from overseas, and their new parents, will have further challenges to face in that the children will not only have been removed from their birth family, but also from their race, language, culture and nationality. Those are huge issues for a child coming to a new country and a new family, and adoptive families need to be supported with dealing with them.

Eligibility for adoption

The child is the most important thing when considering who can and can't adopt. In most cases, the child has spent most of their life in the care system, so first they have been taken from their family for a reason, then they've spent years moving from one foster home to another.

In every case, the priority for the local authority and adoption agency is making sure that the child's adopted family is able to provide them with the stability their lives have been lacking. So the two most important things that adoption agencies look for are health and longevity. These children have dealt with more than enough loss and bereavement in their lives already. Now they need someone who will always be there for them, as much as we can assess that, of course. The parents must have the maximum chances of being around for as long as the child needs them.

Note: At the time of going to print, there were changes going through the legislative process regarding adoption leave and pay that had not yet been finalised.

⇨ The above information is reprinted with kind permission from Adoption UK. Please visit www.adoptionuk.org for further information.

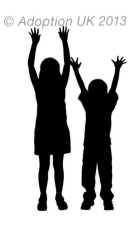

Surrogacy

What is surrogacy?

Surrogacy is when another woman carries and gives birth to a baby for the couple who want to have a child.

The HFEA does not regulate surrogacy. We recommend that you should seek legal advice before proceeding with this option.

Is surrogacy for me?

Surrogacy may be appropriate if you have a medical condition that makes it impossible or dangerous to get pregnant and to give birth.

The type of medical conditions that might make surrogacy necessary for you include:

⇨ absence or malformation of the womb

⇨ recurrent pregnancy loss

⇨ repeated in vitro fertilisation (IVF) implantation failures.

How does surrogacy work?

Full surrogacy (also known as Host or Gestational) – Full surrogacy involves the implantation of an embryo created using either:

⇨ the eggs and sperm of the intended parents

⇨ a donated egg fertilised with sperm from the intended father

⇨ an embryo created using donor eggs and sperm.

Partial surrogacy (also known Straight or Traditional) – Partial surrogacy involves sperm from the intended father and an egg from the surrogate. Here fertilisation is (usually) done by artificial insemination or intrauterine insemination (IUI).

What is my chance of having a baby with surrogacy?

It is quite difficult to determine a success rate for surrogacy, as many factors are relevant, including:

⇨ the surrogate's ability to get pregnant

⇨ the age of the egg donor (if involved)

⇨ the success of procedures such as IUI and IVF

⇨ the quality of gamete provided by the commissioning couple.

The age of the woman who provides the egg is the most important factor that affects chances of pregnancy.

What are the risks of surrogacy?

The risks associated with surrogacy depend on the type of surrogacy (full or partial) undertaken. Generally, the risks associated with full surrogacy are similar to those for IVF.

There is also a risk of transferring HIV and hepatitis, and so screening of everyone involved in surrogacy involving IUI is recommended, and required in surrogacy arrangements involving IVF.

If a registered donor at a licensed clinic is used, the donor will automatically be screened.

Legal issues associated with surrogacy

Surrogacy involves complicated legal issues and we recommend that you seek your own legal advice before making any decisions. It is important to know that surrogacy arrangements are unenforceable.

It is also advisable to receive counselling before starting the surrogacy process, to help you think about all the questions involved.

The rights of the surrogate

You should bear in mind that the surrogate has the legal right to keep the child, even if it is not genetically related to her.

Surrogacy arrangements are not legally enforceable, even if a contract has been signed and the expenses of the surrogate have been paid.

The surrogate will be the legal mother of the child unless or until parenthood is transferred to the intended mother through a parental order or adoption after the birth of the child. This is because, in law, the woman who gives birth is always treated as the mother.

What if the surrogate mother changes her mind?

The surrogate has the legal right to change her mind and keep the child, even when the baby she gave birth to is not genetically related to her. This is difficult for everyone concerned and that's why it is vital that you trust each other and are clear about what is going to happen.

Familiarise yourself with the wording of the Surrogacy Arrangements Act, 1985, or discuss its implications with your lawyer before proceeding.

Clinics have to consider the possibility of a breakdown in the surrogacy arrangements and whether this is likely to cause serious harm to the child to be born or to existing children.

The father's rights

Unless parenthood is transferred to the intended father or second parent through a parental order or adoption:

⇨ the child's legal father or second parent will be the surrogate's husband, civil partner (unless it is shown that husband/civil partner did not consent to the treatment) or partner (if the partner consented to being the father/second parent)

⇨ if treatment was performed in a licensed clinic and the surrogate

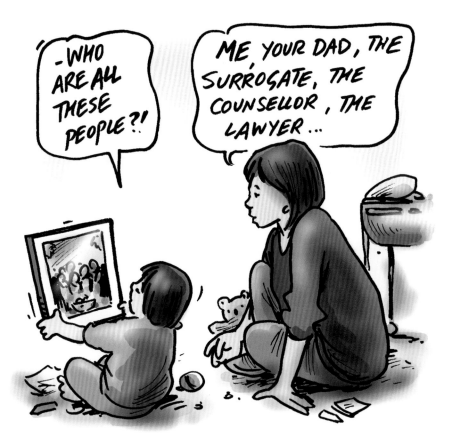

the UK – commercial surrogacy is illegal. However, the intended parents are responsible for the reasonable expenses of the surrogate (for example, clothes, travel expenses and loss of earnings).

Extra expense may be incurred should the surrogate have twins or more.

Clinic surrogacy fees – Fees to the clinic will depend on whether the arrangement involves insemination only or IVF procedures. The fees will also vary depending on which clinic is used and how many attempts you have.

You should ensure that you know the full costs involved before starting surrogacy treatment.

Remember: commercial surrogacy is illegal in the UK – people thinking about surrogacy should be wary of agencies purporting to offer this service.

mother has no partner, the child will have no legal father or second parent.

Becoming the child's legal parents – parental orders

If the intended parents wish to become the legal parents of the child, they may either apply to adopt the child, or apply for a parental order.

The effect of the order is to transfer the rights and obligations of parentage to the intended parents, providing certain conditions are met.

Applications for a parental order must generally be made to the Court within six months of the birth of the child.

To obtain a parental order, at least one of the commissioning couple must be genetically related to the baby i.e. be the egg or sperm provider. Couples must be husband and wife, civil partners or two persons who are living as partners.

Becoming the child's legal parents – adoption

If the commissioning couple cannot apply for a parental order because neither of them are genetically related to the baby (donor egg and

donor sperm or donor embryos were used), then adoption of the baby is the only option available to them.

If adoption is to be the option used, then a registered adoption agency must be involved in the surrogacy process. This is why it is important to get legal advice before you decide to embark on surrogacy.

What happens if the child is born outside the UK?

In a surrogacy arrangement, if the child is born abroad, the commissioning couple can apply for a parental order only if they are living (or domiciled) in the UK.

The parental order officially transfers parental responsibilities to the commissioning couple.

While waiting for the parental order to be processed, the child born abroad will require a visa in order to enter the UK.

If you are considering surrogacy abroad, seek legal advice before going ahead.

Payment issues

Paying surrogate expenses- You are not allowed to pay for a surrogate in

Where do I start?

Once you have decided, in consultation with your fertility specialist, that a surrogacy arrangement is suitable for your circumstances, you must find a surrogate.

Fertility clinics are not allowed to find a surrogate mother for you. There may be unregulated organisations in the UK that may be able to help you – the Infertility Network UK (INUK) may be a good starting point.

You should also be prepared to make the appropriate legal arrangements in order to be recognised in law as the parent of the child.

Choosing a surrogate – You will want to choose a woman capable of having a safe, healthy pregnancy and birth. It is also vital that you build up a trusting relationship with the surrogate.

⇨ The above information is reprinted with kind permission from the Human Fertilisation & Embryology Authority (HFEA). Please visit www.hfea.gov.uk for further information.

India's surrogate mothers are risking their lives. They urgently need protection

As rich westerners flock to India's unregulated baby factories, impoverished surrogates suffer appalling conditions.

By Kishwar Desai

Premila Vaghela, a poor 30-year-old surrogate mother, died last month, while reportedly waiting for a routine examination at a hospital in Ahmedabad. The news was barely covered by the media – after all, she had completed the task she had been contracted for, and the eight-month-old foetus meant for an American 'commissioning' parent survived.

In fact Premila was like many other economically marginalised surrogates, who may suffer or even lose their lives while carrying a child, and are quickly forgotten. The highly secretive and largely unregulated baby factories (many of which are dressed up as legitimate IVF clinics) now mushrooming all over India are usually only concerned with the end product: the child.

Even conservative estimates show more than 25,000 children are now being born through surrogates in India every year in an industry worth $2 billion. These clinics are not just spreading in big cities but in smaller towns as well. Domestic demand is increasing, but as fertility levels drop elsewhere, at least 50% of these babies are 'commissioned' by overseas, mainly western, couples.

Whoever the prospective parents, the pattern is the same: it is only India's desperately poor women who are tempted to rent their wombs. Since the cost of fertility treatment and that of the surrogate is comparatively cheaper in India than in the rest of the world, would-be parents are flooding in, eager to have a child that bears some part of their genetic heritage.

Most of the industry is operating unchecked. India's medical research watchdog drafted regulations more than two years ago, yet they still await presentation in parliament, leaving the surrogates and baby factories open to abuse.

> **"It is only India's desperately poor women who are tempted to rent their wombs"**

And even many of the supposedly well-run clinics do not appear to be transparent in their dealings.

Dr Manish Banker, from the Pulse Women's Hospital, is reported to have said that Premila had come for a check-up. 'She suddenly had a convulsion and fell on the floor,' he said. 'We immediately took her for treatment. Since she was showing signs of distress, we conducted an emergency Caesarean section delivery.'

The child, who was born a month premature, was admitted to the intensive care unit. Premila was moved to another hospital, which claims she was in a highly critical condition, having suffered a cardiac arrest. Although there's no suggestion that this was the case with Premila, sadly, in many cases the surrogate's life is secondary. It is the baby, for whose birth the hospital is being paid, that is paramount.

Most mothers sign contracts agreeing that even if they are seriously injured during the later stages of pregnancy, or suffer any life-threatening illness, they

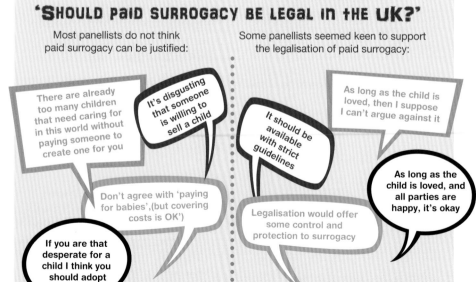

YOUGOV PANELLISTS WERE ASKED:
'SHOULD PAID SURROGACY BE LEGAL IN THE UK?'

Most panellists do not think paid surrogacy can be justified:

There are already too many children that need caring for in this world without paying someone to create one for you

It's disgusting that someone is willing to sell a child

Don't agree with 'paying for babies',(but covering costs is OK')

If you are that desperate for a child I think you should adopt

Some panellists seemed keen to support the legalisation of paid surrogacy:

It should be available with strict guidelines

As long as the child is loved, then I suppose I can't argue against it

As long as the child is loved, and all parties are happy, it's okay

Legalisation would offer some control and protection to surrogacy

Source: Should paid surrogacy be legal? 1 February 2011 © 2000-2013 YouGov plc.

will be 'sustained with life-support equipment' to protect the foetus. Further, they usually agree to assume all medical, financial and psychological risks – releasing the genetic parents, their lawyers, the doctors and all other professionals from all liabilities.

Besides, in tragic cases like Premila's, the hospital would have quickly paid out the money owed for a 'successful' birth, so the family would be unlikely to complain. Premila herself had gone in for the surrogacy to provide her own two children a better life. In a country where thousands of women die every year in normal childbirths, who would complain about the death of one surrogate?

Anindita Majumdar, who is researching surrogacy for her doctorate, says she is personally distressed by how easily the 'sheer horror' of it all is being swept away by the money paid out to the surrogates. There are many grey areas – and she fears that even the draft legislation, when it is passed, will favour the medical community over the rights of the surrogate.

Already many malpractices, such as implantation of more than four embryos in the surrogate's womb, as well as invasive 'foetal reduction' frowned on the world over, are being followed. Often women undergo caesareans so the time of birth suits the commissioning parents.

While researching my novel I found that women are more than willing to undergo the risks. They feel that by renting their wombs (perhaps the only asset they possess), they can make enough money to look after their families. And indeed, many have earned enough to build small homes for their families, and buy some security for their children's schooling. One surrogate told me she wanted her daughter to receive a proper education and speak English just like I did. She was only 21, and carrying twins for a commissioning couple – but she was already planning her next three surrogacies.

One woman, according to another researcher, had over 20 cycles of hormonal injections. Since each child is often born through Caesarean section (so that the birth coincides with the arrival of the commissioning parents) the health of the surrogate is likely to suffer with each operation.

I found that medical practitioners involved in it are rarely troubled about the fate of the women whose normal maternal cycles have been disrupted. As in Premila's case, they seem to be only interested in delivering the end-product: a child.

If India doesn't pass the regulatory bill soon, the international community should pressurise it to do so. This is now a global industry so requires an international law and a global fertility body to regulate it. Otherwise, it is likely that most of the unhealthy practices prevailing will go underground – and the fog of secrecy over the industry will become more dense.

5 June 2012

⇨ The above information is reprinted with kind permission from The Guardian. Please visit www.guardian.co.uk for further information.

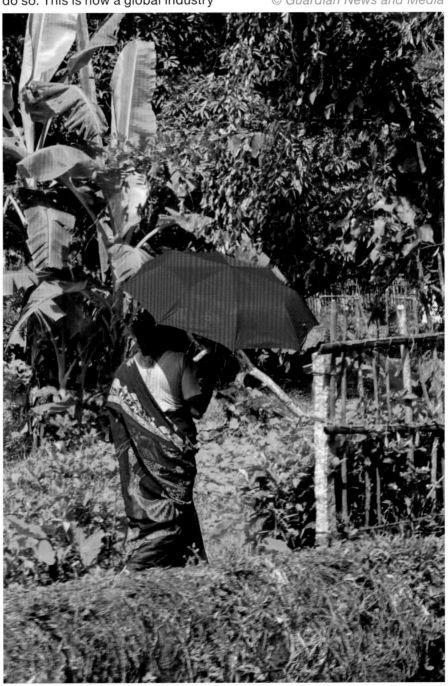

Greater treatment options for women with fertility problems

More women can receive appropriate and timely fertility treatment such as IVF, following updated guidelines from NICE.

Infertility is a common medical condition which can have devastating, painful, and life-long effects extending to personal relationships and wider family.

It is caused by various reasons, with a quarter of cases unexplained, a further quarter caused by ovulatory disorders, and 30 per cent of cases due to factors affecting male fertility.

The condition affects around one in seven heterosexual couples, with both the number of people affected by fertility problems, and those seeking help for them, increasing over the past decade.

The rising number of people seeking help coincides with an increasing trend for couples to start families

later in life, despite fertility declining rapidly with age, especially after 35. In 2011, women who received fertility treatment were 35 years old on average, and had been trying to conceive for around four years.

NICE has updated its guidelines on fertility to ensure people experiencing fertility problems get the most appropriate and effective treatment earlier.

In the previous 2004 fertility guideline, NICE said that IVF treatment should not be recommended for women older than 39.

Under the updated recommendations, NICE says that under certain criteria, women aged between 40 and 42 years should be offered one full cycle of IVF with or without intracytoplasmic sperm, if they have not conceived after two years of regular unprotected intercourse, or 12 cycles of artificial insemination where six or more are by intrauterine insemination.

The definition of a full cycle of IVF has been updated to prevent any ambiguity in interpretation or variation in treatment. A full cycle is now defined as including one episode of ovarian stimulation and the transfer of any resultant fresh and frozen embryos.

The updated guideline also recommends that IVF treatment should be made available for eligible women earlier than was previously recommended.

Women who are eligible for IVF can now receive treatment after two years of regular vaginal intercourse, or 12 cycles of artificial insemination, if they have been unable to conceive. This is one year earlier than in the previous recommendations.

The updated guideline additionally contains recommendations to ensure that only the most effective treatments are offered in a timely manner to people experiencing problems in conceiving.

NICE says people with unexplained infertility, mild endometriosis or mild male factor infertility should attempt to conceive through regular vaginal intercourse for two years rather than receive intrauterine insemination.

This is because evidence available since the previous guideline was published shows that intrauterine insemination treatment provides no further benefit to producing a live birth than regular vaginal intercourse.

Furthermore, oral ovarian stimulation agents, such as clomefine citrate, anastrozole or letrozole, should now not be offered to women with unexplained fertility.

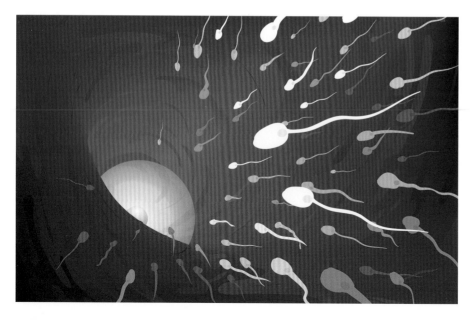

The guideline for the first time also covers same-sex couples, those who carry infectious diseases such as Hepatitis B or HIV, and those who are unable to have intercourse, for example if they have a physical disability.

Tim Child, a Consultant Gynaecologist and Director of the Oxford Fertility Unit and member of the Guideline Development Group, said: 'Recommending IVF treatment for a very select group of women over 40 was not a decision that was taken lightly. When a woman reaches her mid-30s her fertility begins to decline, even more so from her late 30s.

'However, many women do conceive naturally in the 40–42 year age group, but for those who can't, and who have been diagnosed with the medical condition of infertility, then improvement in IVF success rates over the last decade mean that we are now able to offer cost-effective treatment with a single IVF cycle.'

He added: 'This decision was taken after considerable discussion and close analysis of the available evidence.'

Sir Andrew Dillon, Chief Executive of NICE, said: 'Whatever the cause, we know fertility problems can have a potentially devastating effect on people's lives; causing significant distress, depression and possibly leading to the breakdown of relationships.

'The good news is that, thanks to a number of medical advances over the years, many fertility problems can be treated effectively.

'It is because of these new advances that we have been able to update our guideline on fertility, ensuring that the right support, care and treatment is available to those who will benefit the most.'

20 February 2013

⇨ National Institute for Health and Clinical Excellence (2013). Greater treatment options for women with fertility problems. London: NICE. Available at www.nice.org.uk. Reproduced with permission.

Women over 40 should be offered IVF on the NHS, board suggests

Women aged 40–42 who are having fertility problems should be offered IVF on the NHS, according to guidelines published on Wednesday by the National Institute for Health and Clinical Excellence (NICE).

Previously, NICE did not recommend IVF for women older than 39.

The guidelines also recommend IVF treatment for eligible women who have been unable to conceive after two years of regular intercourse – one year earlier than previously recommended.

They also cover women who have been having artificial insemination, which can include same-sex couples. This is the first time these have been officially included in the guidelines, which were originally drawn up in 2004.

The guidelines say women aged 40–42 who have not conceived after two years of regular unprotected intercourse or 12 cycles of artificial insemination should be offered one full cycle of IVF, if they have never previously had IVF treatment.

Where women are under 40, and have not conceived after two years of regular intercourse or 12 cycles of artificial insemination, three cycles of IVF should be offered.

NICE chief executive Sir Andrew Dillon said: 'Infertility affects more people than you might think; around one in seven heterosexual couples in the UK.

'We know fertility problems can have a potentially devastating effect on people's lives, causing significant distress, depression and possibly leading to the breakdown of relationships.

'The good news is that, thanks to a number of medical advances over the years, many fertility problems can be treated effectively.

'It is because of these new advances that we have been able to update our guideline on fertility, ensuring that the right support, care and treatment is available to those who will benefit the most.'

Tim Child, consultant gynaecologist and director of the Oxford Fertility Unit, who helped develop the guidelines, said: 'Many women do conceive naturally in the 40–42 year age group, but for those who can't, and who have been diagnosed with the medical condition of infertility, then improvement in IVF success rates over the last decade mean that we are now able to offer cost

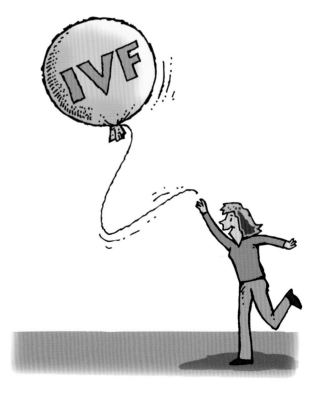

effective treatment with a single IVF cycle.

'This decision was taken after considerable discussion and close analysis of the available evidence.'

On same-sex couples, a spokeswoman for NICE said: 'With the advancement of medical technology and techniques such as donor insemination, same-sex couples are now able to become parents.

'Infertility is a medical condition that can be caused by a past illness or underlying medical condition and can affect anyone, regardless of sexual orientation. Infertility can also cause real suffering and can lead to depression and the break-down of relationships.

'This is the first time same-sex couples have been included in NICE guidance on fertility. In terms of fertility treatment, same-sex couples only account for a small proportion of NHS patients – around 5%.

'However, it is important that we are sure that everyone who has this distressing medical condition has access to the best levels of help.'

A full cycle of fresh IVF can cost the NHS around £3,000.

The National Infertility Awareness Campaign (NIAC) warned that as NICE guidelines are not mandatory, fears still remained over local implementation.

Chairwoman Clare Lewis-Jones said: 'By updating the fertility guideline and extending the range of people it is recommending receive treatment, NICE clearly understands the impact which infertility has on people. And we must be clear that infertility is a medical condition that causes significant distress for those trying to have a baby and has a devastating impact on people's lives.

'We know infertility can be treated effectively and thousands of people have become parents after fertility treatment.

'The current "postcode lottery" approach to the treatment of infertility here has gone on for far too long and it is vital that the Government supports the measures in the updated guideline and communicates the need to implement them to those who commission fertility services in the NHS.

'We know the current system leaves many people unable to access NHS treatment and we need reassurance about the future of NHS fertility treatment as we move towards GP commissioning in 2013.

'The new guideline gives hope to more infertility sufferers – but it is pointless if the recommendations are not put into practice. People are suffering every day because some PCTs have continually flouted the NICE guideline.

'Infertility requires specialist knowledge and GPs are, by their very definition, generalists.

'Over 50% of respondents to our patient survey last year found their GP lacked sufficient knowledge on infertility and this worries us.

'NIAC is willing and able to work with the Government to close this knowledge gap so that access to fertility treatment is improved in the new NHS.'

The Royal College of Obstetricians and Gynaecologists said the new guidelines offered more choice to women trying to conceive up to the age of 42.

President Dr Tony Falconer said: 'We welcome the updated guidelines and support that people experiencing fertility problems should be able to get the most appropriate and effective medical treatment and in a timely fashion.'

He added: 'We strongly endorse the recommendation that single embryo transfer is used if possible for women aged 39 and under. We know that replacing more than one embryo in the uterus can result in a multiple pregnancy, which carries a higher risk of complications, therefore a reduction in multiple births would have major benefits to both mother and child.

'We are aware that maternal age has risen over the years and that it is harder for older women to conceive naturally. The recommendation that IVF treatment be made available up to the age of 42 provides more choice for women but they should still be aware of the increased risks associated with pregnancy at advanced maternal age.'

20 February 2013

⇨ The above information is reprinted with kind permission from *The Huffington Post UK*, which is provided by AOL (UK) Limited. Please visit www. huffingtonpost.co.uk for further information.

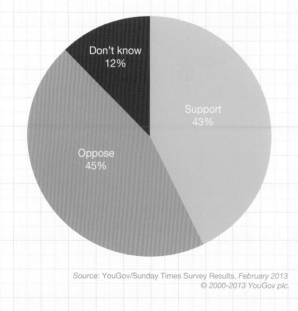

NHS guidelines for IVF treatment for people unable to have children have been changed to increase the maximum age for IVF treatment from 39 to 42. Do you support or oppose this change?

Don't know 12%

Support 43%

Oppose 45%

Source: YouGov/Sunday Times Survey Results, *February 2013*
© 2000-2013 YouGov plc.

Columnist questions NHS funding IVF for over-40s

A national newspaper columnist has questioned the wisdom of the NHS funding IVF for over 40s – following draft guidance which recommended such a move.

Writing as a woman who knows 'what it's like to be desperate for a child', Amanda Platell warned that the idea of giving free IVF to some women up to the age of 42 is not only wasteful but also cruel.

In her column she also suggested the reason some people put off having children is because they pursued other goals earlier in life.

Sadness

And she says the 'cash-strapped' NHS should not be diverting its resources from other needs.

The columnist described how she had experienced the 'envy of seeing friends deliver another child effortlessly' and the sadness of wishing she was able to buy baby clothes for her own child and not someone else's.

But she said that after a series of operations and a decade of trying, she had to face the 'reality' that being a mother was not an 'entitlement'.

However she added: 'I spent my own hard-earned cash paying for my treatment', because she thought it was wrong for the state to pay.

Warn

Amanda Platell also warned about the 'terrible cycle of hope and despair' for older women having IVF, and noted that it often does not lead to pregnancy for women over 40.

The commentator wrote that some women focus on jobs, homes and luxuries before getting to 40 and realising that they want a baby.

But she said taxpayers should not have to 'fork out millions of pounds for the lifestyle choices' of these women.

Too late

The columnist commented that many are 'putting off motherhood until their 40s' because of a 'decision to pursue their own lives and happiness and let motherhood wait until they're ready'.

'Too often by then it is too late, which is terribly sad. But if these women really were so driven by their maternal instincts, they wouldn't have left it two decades, would they?', she concluded.

25 May 2012

⇨ The above information is reprinted with kind permission from The Christian Institute. Please visit www.christian.org.uk for further information.

IVF mum, 57, now admits: 'I'm too old'

By Carolyn Robertson

When Susan Tollefsen conceived via in vitro fertilisation at the age of 57, it was a dream come true – despite the public criticism. Three years later, as a 61-year-old single mum to a toddler, she now agrees that there should be an upper age limit on child-bearing.

'If I'm completely honest, my experience has taught me that 50 should probably be the cut-off limit for having children, but until you have them it's almost impossible to appreciate that,' Susan reveals. 'It's so true that you only learn by your own mistakes, and my mistake was not to have had her sooner.'

Freya was conceived using a donor egg and the sperm of Susan's then partner Nick Mayer. Though the pair were in a committed relationship at the time of their daughter's birth, the pressures of parenting soon caused a rift: 'I felt as if he didn't want his family life to change at all after Freya came along, even though mine had changed completely,' says Susan.

Though she insists that her daughter is 'without doubt the best thing I have ever done in my life', Susan adds, 'My mistake was not to have had her sooner.'

It's more than just the day-to-day demands of motherhood that have opened Susan's eyes; the prospect of not being able to watch Freya grow up haunts her.

'I get a great emotional feeling when I look at her and a sadness when I realise that time's running out. If I could change just one thing I would wish to be younger so I could enjoy watching Freya grow up, get married and have children of her own,' Susan says. 'I'm doing my best to raise her to be completely independent but the prospect of her being taken from me, if I die, particularly when she's still young, breaks my heart.'

Susan's confession comes on the heels of last week's news that more and more women are putting off parenthood, with new data showing that the number of births for women 50 and older has risen 300% since 1997.

7 November 2011

⇨ The above information is reproduced with kind permission from babycenter.com. Please visit www.babycenter.com for further information.

IVF: the older women who have become mothers

Women could remain fertile indefinitely after successful ovarian transplants lead to births and delay the menopause, doctors have told a conference. Here are the women who have become mothers later in life following IVF.

By Hannah Furness

In 2008, Susan Tollefsen successfully conceived after receiving IVF treatment from a Russian clinic aged 57. She and partner Nick Mayer, who was 11 years her junior, went on to have a baby girl named Freya. At the time, she said: 'I'm still so full of life and healthy at 60 I don't see any reason why I shouldn't be treated.' After originally defending her decision, she last year admitted she had difficulties as an older mother and advocated an age limit of 50 for IVF treatment.

In 2009, 66-year-old Elizabeth Adeney gave birth to a son in Cambridge, following IVF treatment in Ukraine. When asked about her IVF treatments, Mrs Adeney said: 'It's not physical age that is important – it's how I feel inside. Some days I feel 39. Others, I feel 56.' She planned to raise her son as a single mother.

In 2006, psychiatrist Patricia Rashbrook, from Lewes, East Sussex, gave birth to a son when she was 62 years old. She and her husband John had travelled to the former Soviet Republic, where she underwent IVF treatment. Her son, named Jay Jay, was born by Caesarean section at the Sussex County Hospital. At the time, the IVF specialist who treated her said: 'Age isn't important in this decision – what's important is the physical condition of the mother.'

In 2006, Maria del Carmen Bousada de Lara gave birth to twin sons, Pau and Christian, at Sant Pau Hospital in Barcelona, Spain, just one week before her 67th birthday. She had travelled to America for treatment, allegedly lying about her age. The babies were delivered prematurely by Caesarean section and weighed 3.5 lb each. She died from stomach cancer when her sons were two-and-a-half years old. She had previously argued that there was no reason to believe she would not have as long a life as her mother, who died at the age of 101, and joked that she might live to see her grandchildren.

In 2008, Rajo Devi Lohan gave birth to daughter Naveen aged 70 after receiving IVF in India. When her daughter was just 18 months old, Mrs Lohan revealed she was dying after failing to recover from complications after surgery. She said: 'I dreamed about having a child all my life. It does not matter to me that I am ill, because at least I lived long enough to become a mother.'

In July 2008, 70-year-old Omkari Panwar gave birth to twins by emergency Caesarean section in hospital in Muzaffarnagar, India. The twins, a boy and a girl, were born a month premature and weighing 2lb each. Her 77-year-old husband said: 'The treatment cost me a fortune but the birth of a son makes it all worthwhile. I can die a happy man and a proud father.'

In 2010, Bhateri Devi gave birth to triplets, two boys and a girl, in Haryana, India at the age of 66. She is the oldest known woman to give birth to triplets and underwent IVF treatment. She already had two daughters but was desperate for a male heir.

5 July 2012

⇨ The above information is reprinted with kind permission from *The Telegraph*. Please visit www.telegraph.co.uk for further information.

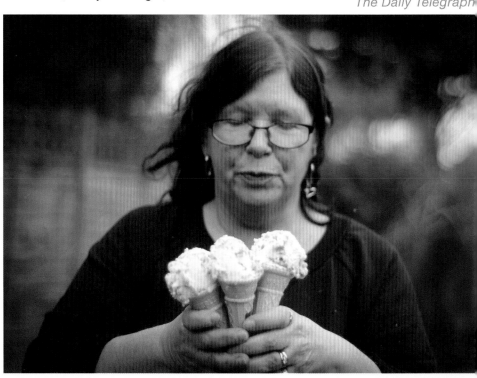

UK: anti-abortion group claims extending IVF to gay couples is 'social engineering'

By Scott Roberts

The Society for the Protection of Unborn Children has denounced plans to provide gay couples with greater access to IVF treatment and says it amounts to 'politically correct social engineering'.

The National Institute for Health and Clinical Excellence (NICE) is expected to make the recommendations in a report this week.

"Same-sex couples have chosen a naturally non-fertile lifestyle and we shouldn't be spending millions of pounds of taxpayers' money on them"

NICE will recommend that same-sex couples be offered artificial insemination on the NHS for six cycles before moving on to IVF if that fails.

Anthony Ozimic, communications manager for the Society for the Protection of Unborn Children (SPUC), an anti-abortion lobby group, criticised the new guidelines. He said: 'This decision ignores biology in the face of politically correct social engineering.

'Same-sex couples do not have fertility problems, they have chosen a naturally non-fertile lifestyle, and we shouldn't be spending millions of pounds of taxpayers' money on fertility procedures for people who do not have fertility problems.'

However, James Taylor, health officer for gay rights charity Stonewall, dismissed the SPUC's claims. 'There is no research that shows being brought up by two dads or two mums puts you in any worse position than being brought up by a mum and a dad,' said Mr Taylor.

Last October, the SPUC attacked proposals to legalise same-sex marriage in England and Wales at a conference in Blackpool.

John Smeaton, director of the society, said: 'Marriage will be undermined

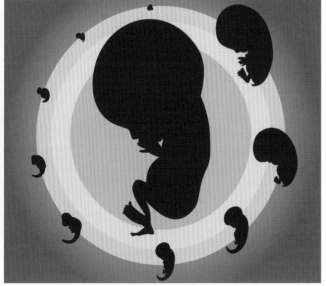

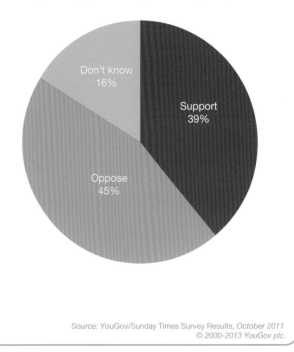

Currently, people who donate sperm or eggs for infertility treatments can only be paid expenses. It has been proposed that payments up to £750 should be allowed to encourage more donations.

Would you support or oppose this policy?

Don't know 16%

Support 39%

Oppose 45%

Source: YouGov/Sunday Times Survey Results, October 2011
© 2000-2013 YouGov plc.

because we will no longer be able to teach our children that marriage exists to protect them.

'If this goes ahead the child will no longer be regarded as fundamental to the married state, marriage will become a genderless institution'.

18 February 2013

⇨ The above information is reproduced with kind permission from Pink News. Please visit www.pinknews.co.uk for further information.

Challenge to landmark ruling on sex offender's right to IVF (poll)

Should a woman be allowed to undergo IVF, if her partner has been convicted of a sexual offence?

According to a patient review panel in Australia, who are challenging a landmark ruling to allow a convicted sex offender's wife to undergo fertility treatment, the answer should be No.

The panel is urging the Court of Appeal to quash a Victorian Civil and Administrative Tribunal (VCAT) decision last year that overturned an automatic ban on IVF access, arising from the sex offender's conviction.

According to *The Herald Sun*, the landmark hearing last year gave the green light to an unnamed sex offender to proceed with the costly IVF treatment, despite a 12-month jail sentence for his crime.

The 34-year-old man and his wife had started the IVF treatment, but were banned from continuing after he was convicted of a sexual offence in 2009.

The Patient Review Panel originally denied the couple access to the treatment in 2010 once he had served his sentence, citing the new Assisted Reproductive Treatment Act as the reason. This act bans criminals from fertility treatment.

However, the Victorian Civil and Administrative Tribunal overturned the decision in 2011, claiming that the man posed no serious danger to minors.

'It is important to appreciate that the purpose of this review is not to further punish (the man) for his offending – a just punishment has already been imposed by the County Court,' then VCAT president Justice Iain Ross ruled, reports *The Herald Sun*.

The Patients Review Panel appealed this ruling today and are hoping to overturn the ruling in the Supreme Court.

Explaining their reasons behind the appeal, Kerri Judd from the Patient Review Panel has said that their focus is not on the man reoffending, but of the best interest in the unborn child.

'What we want is for the correct test to be applied,' Judd told *The Australian*.

'Whatever test is formulated the focus needs to be on the interest of the child.'

16 July 2012

⇨ The above information is reprinted with kind permission from *The Huffington Post UK*, which is provided by AOL (UK) Limited. Visit www.huffingtonpost.co.uk for further information.

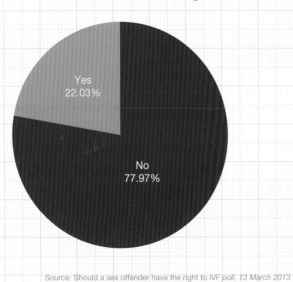

Should a sex offender have the right to IVF?

Yes
22.03%

No
77.97%

Some comments from The Huffington Post's readers:

'Sex offender is too broad a term to just categorically deny all sex offenders the right to IVF. It should be up to a court and a judge each time.'

'If your partner is a sex offender you in my opinion have no right IVF. End of.'

'The question should be whether a sex offender's SPOUSE should be allowed IVF. The spouse is innocent and should be treated as such.'

'The question here is "will a sex offender make a good parent?" No, they won't.'

'Not all sex offenders are child molesters. How do we differentiate between levels of offenders?'

'What a stupid question. More stereotyping of se offenders. Sad.'

'Three-parent IVF' could combat genetic disease

Thousands of people could benefit from a funding boost for research into defective mitochondria – but there are ethical questions, Channel 4 News hears.

In addition to £4.4 million funding from the Wellcome Trust to set up a new research centre at Newcastle University, the Government has announced that it will carry out a consultation on the research, which would ultimately need a change in the law to proceed to the clinic.

The work aims to prevent genetic diseases caused by defective mitochondria – the 'batteries' that power the cells in our bodies. When these fail, patients can develop devastating diseases, with symptoms often affecting tissues such as the heart, muscles and brain. At least one in 5,000 adults is affected by diseases caused in this way.

Now scientists at Newcastle University believe they have found a way to prevent these mitochondrial diseases, which are passed on by the mother to the child. The technique involves replacing the defective mitochondria in a human egg, either before or after it has been fertilised, with healthy mitochondria.

> **"This is something that blights generations of families, and if we can stop that happening it would be incredible"**
>
> *Nicola Bardett, who has a form of mitochondrial disease*

The first technique, known as 'pronuclear transfer', involves taking two fertilised eggs, one from the affected woman, the second from a donor. The researchers remove the nuclear DNA – the part of a cell which contains our genetic make-up – from the donor egg, leaving behind the healthy mitochondria, and replace it with the nucleus from the mother's egg. This new egg is then implanted in the affected woman's womb using IVF. The second technique, known as 'metaphase spindle transfer', involves using non-fertilised eggs at the outset but then fertilising them once the mother's DNA has been transplanted into a healthy donor cell.

This has lead to the method being branded as 'three-parent IVF', raising fears of cloning and other ethical questions.

Patient tests

The technique works in the laboratory, but the Human Fertilisation and Embryology Authority (HFEA) has requested further experiments to assess the technique's safety before it can be accepted and safely used in clinics for patients.

The Government has also asked the HFEA to carry out a consultation to inform the public about mitochondrial disease and to seek its opinion about the use of these methods to avoid such diseases.

Professor Doug Turnbull and Professor Mary Herbert, from Newcastle University, are leading the research and will continue at the new centre at Newcastle University, funded by the Wellcome Trust and £1.4 million from the university itself.

Professor Turnbull said: 'Every year, we see hundreds of patients whose lives are seriously affected by mitochondrial diseases... This new funding will enable us to take forward essential experiments which we hope will demonstrate to the HFEA and to the public that these techniques, which are based on existing IVF techniques, are safe and effective.'

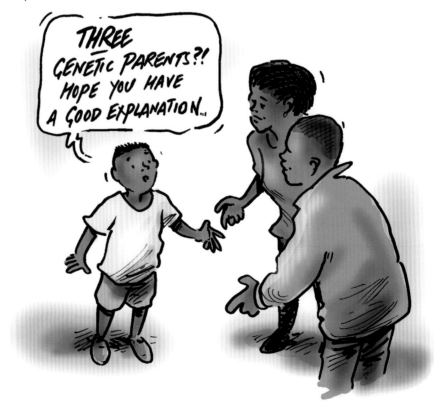

'Serious ethical problems'

While scientists believe that the research could help many thousands of people, there are some people who have concerns over what the process involves.

Helen Watt is senior research director at the Anscombe Centre for Bioethics in Oxford, a Roman Catholic academic institute. She told Channel 4 News that both the techniques being assessed by the HFEA involve 'very serious ethical problems'.

Regarding pronuclear transfer, she said: 'This grossly disrespects human life, and any child born from this particular technique will sadly discover she has no genetic parents – not three parents, as is sometimes reported. Instead, she is formed from the bodies of two embryos created and killed precisely as 'building blocks' for hers.

'We are very far here from the unconditional welcome of new life which having a baby should involve.'

She added: 'Even with the second, less destructive method, maternal spindle transfer, where nuclear material is exchanged before fertilisation, the child will face the unknown physical risks of the procedure in addition to the identity problems of knowing she that has, in this case, three genetic parents. For couples who, understandably, do not want to take the risk of passing on mitochondrial disorders to their children, adoption is a far better solution.'

19 January 2012

⇨ The above information is reprinted with kind permission from Channel 4. Please visit www.channel4.com for further information.

'Incredible'

Nicola Bardett, 33, from Northumberland has a form of mitochondrial disease called Melas syndrome. Many people in her family also have the condition, including her mother, who died at 52. Nicola will also pass the condition on to her children. She has a three-year-old son.

'My mum started to show symptoms on and off from around the age of 19, then she just steadily got worse and worse. She started to go deaf when she was 35. By the time she died she was like an old woman and had started to develop dementia in the year before she died,' she said.

'Although I don't have any symptoms yet myself, this still has a massive impact on my life and on the lives of everyone in our family. It is like a ticking time-bomb that could strike at any time... When I had my son, we didn't realise the full implications of carrying this defect.

'If this work is allowed to go ahead it could wipe out this problem from future generations. This is something that blights generation after generation of families and if we can stop that happening it would be incredible.'

How does three parent IVF work?

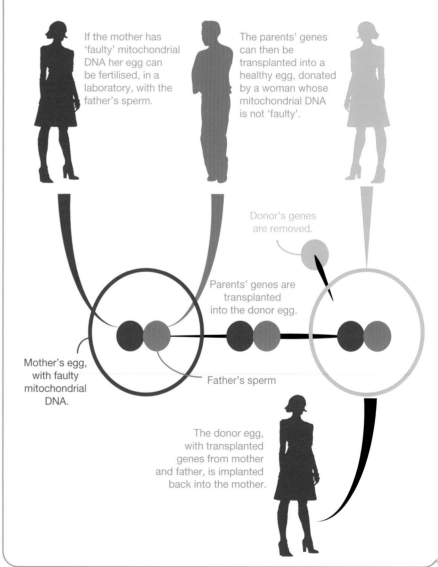

If the mother has 'faulty' mitochondrial DNA her egg can be fertilised, in a laboratory, with the father's sperm.

The parents' genes can then be transplanted into a healthy egg, donated by a woman whose mitochondrial DNA is not 'faulty'.

Donor's genes are removed.

Parents' genes are transplanted into the donor egg.

Mother's egg, with faulty mitochondrial DNA.

Father's sperm

The donor egg, with transplanted genes from mother and father, is implanted back into the mother.

Ethical committee finds IVF by three parents morally justified

A report from an influential think tank could help clear the way to IVF babies being born with DNA from three different people.

By Sarah O'Meara

Outlawed techniques that give a baby DNA from a father, a mother and a woman donor to prevent inherited disorders are morally justified, says the Nuffield Council on Bioethics.

Their purpose is to stop the transmission of defective mitochondrial DNA (mDNA) from mothers to their babies.

Children born after the procedures would possess nuclear DNA inherited from their parents plus mitochondrial DNA (mDNA) from a woman donor.

Mitochondria are rod-shaped power plants in the bodies of cells that supply energy. They contain their own DNA, which is only passed down the maternal line.

Faulty mitochondrial genes can lead to a wide range of serious disorders including heart malfunction, kidney and liver disease, stroke, dementia and blindness, as well as premature death.

Around 6,000 adults in the UK are believed to be affected by mitochondrial diseases.

Controversy surrounds attempts to prevent such diseases through hi-tech variations of In-Vitro Fertilisation (IVF) treatment.

One technique, pronuclear transfer, involves transferring nuclear DNA out of a day-old embryonic cell containing defective mitochondria. The DNA is planted into another single-cell embryo whose mitochondria function normally.

The donor embryo's own nuclear DNA is discarded. However, it still contains the normal mitochondria of the woman whose egg was fertilised to create it.

As it grows, the embryo produces a baby with DNA from three sources – nuclear DNA from the original parents, plus a tiny amount of mitochondrial DNA from the woman egg donor.

Another technique, maternal spindle transfer (MST), is similar but involves transferring nuclear DNA from an unfertilised egg to a donor egg. The egg is then fertilised using the father's sperm.

Although such techniques are banned, they could be voted in by Parliament under existing legislation.

A working group of the Nuffield Council on Bioethics decided that such treatments would be ethical, despite tampering with inherited DNA.

Although mDNA has important biological effects, it is not believed to have any impact on basic individual characteristics.

Dr Geoff Watts, who chaired the Council inquiry, said: 'If further research shows these techniques to be sufficiently safe and effective, we think it would be ethical for families to use them if they wished to, provided they receive an appropriate level of information and support.

'They could offer significant health and social benefits to individuals and families, who could potentially live their lives free from what can be very severe and debilitating disorders.

'We would recommend that families commit to allowing long-term follow-up of the resulting children, supported by a centrally-funded register of such procedures performed in the UK, which would be accessible to researchers over several decades.'

He added: 'We understand that some people concerned about the idea of germline therapies may fear that if such treatments for mitochondrial gene disorders were approved, a 'slippery slope' would be created towards comparable alterations to the nuclear genome.

'However, we are only talking about the use of these techniques in the clearly-defined situation of otherwise incurable mitochondrial disorders, under strict regulation.'

Professor Frances Flinter, a clinical geneticist and member of the working group, pointed out that only 0.1% of affected children's DNA would be donated.

'As far as we know, mitochondrial genes alone create no unique identifiable genetic link between the child and donor,' she said.

'The child's recognisable likeness to family members would come from their parents' nuclear DNA. Given these, and other reasons, we think it is both legally and biologically inaccurate to refer to a mitochondrial donor as a 'second mother' or 'third parent' to the child.'

Anthony Ozimic, spokesman for the pro-life group Society for the Protection of Unborn Children (SPUC) said: 'As with IVF and cloning, this mitochondrial technique may well lead to the developmental abnormalities. Creating embryonic children in the laboratory abuses them, by subjecting them to unnatural processes. These techniques are both destructive and dangerous and therefore unethical.

'The vast majority of embryonic children created in the laboratory are killed because they do not meet the 'quality control' requirements dictated by scientists involved in such increasingly macabre experiments.

'Scientists should abandon the spurious field of destructive embryo experimentation and instead promote the ethical alternative of adult stem cell research, which is already providing cures and treatments for an increasing number of conditions.'

A statement from the Human Fertilisation and Embryology Authority, which regulates fertility treatment and research, said: 'The HFEA welcomes this timely and important report from the Nuffield Council on Bioethics. We share the Council's belief that continuing public debate about these issues is important; the HFEA will lead this debate.

'We will launch a public consultation in September 2012, as part of a wider programme of public engagement throughout the year. Our aim is to facilitate a lively and informed debate in order to gauge public perceptions of the ethical and social issues surrounding the use of IVF techniques designed to prevent mitochondrial disease in treatment. We will report our findings to Ministers in Spring 2013.'

Dr David King, director of the group Human Genetics Alert, accused scientists of acting like 'Frankenstein'.

He said: 'The proposed techniques are both unnecessary and highly dangerous in the medium term, since they set a precedent for allowing the creation of genetically modified designer babies. But these considerations are ignored by the bioethics industry because of its flawed methodology and in its usual rush to embrace risky hi-tech 'solutions'.'

Dr King added: 'What worries most people about constructing a person in this way is the same thing that worries them about GM foods or human animal hybrids: the way that scientists treat nature as a set of infinitely exchangeable parts to be mixed and matched as necessary.

'Just as Frankenstein's creation was produced by sticking together bits from many different bodies, it seems that there is no grotesquerie, no violation of the norms of nature or human culture at which scientists and their bioethical helpers will balk. But such concerns cannot be admitted as real within the discourse of bioethics and can certainly never overcome its trump cards of 'medical progress' or simply 'increasing knowledge'.'

12 June 2012

⇨ The above information is reprinted with kind permission from *The Huffington Post UK*, which is provided by AOL (UK) Limited. Please visit www.huffingtonpost.co.uk for further information.

HFEA launches public consultation on 'three parent' IVF technique

Authority tests public temperature on mitochondria replacement.

The Human Fertilisation & Embryology Authority has launched a public consultation on the ethics of new IVF-based techniques designed to avoid serious mitochondrial diseases.

Around one in 200 children are born each year with a form of mitochondrial disease. Some children have mild or no symptoms but others can be severely affected and have a shortened life expectancy. Symptoms include muscle weakness, intestinal disorders and heart disease.

New techniques, known as mitochondria replacement (and labelled by some 'three parent IVF'), could enable women to avoid passing these diseases on to their children by using a donor's mitochondria to create a healthy embryo, which would then be used in normal IVF treatment. Any child born following mitochondria replacement would share DNA with three people, albeit a tiny amount with the donor. These changes would affect the germ line, meaning the donor's mitochondrial DNA would be passed onto future generations.

Mitochondria replacement is currently lawful in the laboratory, but the embryos cannot be used in treatment. The Government has asked the HFEA, as the expert independent regulator, to seek public views on whether these techniques should be made available to couples at risk of having an affected child.

Chair of the HFEA, Professor Lisa Jardine said:

'The Government has asked us to take the public temperature on this important and emotive issue.

'The decision about whether mitochondria replacement should be made available to treat patients is not only an issue of great importance to families affected by these terrible diseases, but is also one of enormous public interest. We find ourselves in uncharted territory, balancing the desire to help families have healthy children with the possible impact on the children themselves and wider society.

'We will use our considerable experience of explaining complicated areas of science and ethics to the public to generate a rich debate that is open to all.'

The HFEA has launched an accessible and interactive consultation website, which explains the science and ethical issues in different ways – including videos and downloadable 'discussion packs'. Anyone will be able to register their views online or attend one of two free consultation events in November. More information is available on the HFEA website (www.hfea.gov.uk).

⇨ The above information is reprinted with kind permission from the Human Fertilisation & Embryology Authority (HFEA). Please visit www.hfea.gov.uk for further information.

The big question: are GM babies wrong?

The public is being asked one of the most testing ethical questions it has faced for a generation: should scientists be able to tinker with the building blocks of humanity?

By Zoe and Steve Vaughan

A highly significant medical breakthrough means that children can now be born without mitochondrial diseases, which include a form of muscular dystrophy, vision, hearing and heart problems and intestinal disorders.

Using a procedure which has been dubbed three-parent IVF, scientists are able to remove the unhealthy mitochondria, the 'motors' that power living cells but can cause these problems, and replace them with healthy mitochondria from a donor.

The public is now being asked to say whether they think this super IVF procedure should be allowed or not.

Opponents say we must not mess with millennia of evolution. They say monkeying with the germline – the cells that carry the genetic material – could have terrible consequences for future generations.

The children created will suffer identity crises, it's not natural and it is just the start of a slippery slope that will lead to designer babies. In addition, it will only benefit about ten to 20 couples a year.

Those in favour say science must be allowed to move forward and help save lives. This could be the beginning of a new branch of medicine that stops disease at birth.

All scientific breakthroughs require a leap of faith: the first heart and lung transplant, chemotherapy, laser eye surgery. Now these are routine procedures at hospitals across the country.

The Human Fertilisation and Embryology Authority has given the public until 7 December to comment on the ethics of the procedure.

So we ask: should genetic engineering of babies be banned?

Zoe: No – science can help reduce suffering

All too often the tough bioethical discussions like these can be drowned out by too much thin-end-of-the-wedge shrieking.

In the case of three-parent IVF, as this process has been short-handed, the argument goes that this is simply a development that will pave the way for all-singing, all-dancing designer baby clinics where you sit down select eye/hair/skin colour over a latte and muffin.

Consider then that the fat end of the wedge here is not actually cosmetic child solutions but a branch of medical science that doesn't treat or even cure disease, but prevents it at birth.

Instead of a 'thin end', this could be the cornerstone of a development in medical science that today is about stopping relatively rare diseases but tomorrow could be about stopping inherited cancers.

Before we start getting into the realms of 'it's not natural', let's be clear here: most of medical science isn't. Hearts are supposed to stop beating, not be restarted, regulated by pacemakers and transplanted. If we are to let nature take its course rather than fight it with science, then are we to give up seeking cures for cancer, motor neurone disease and Parkinson's?

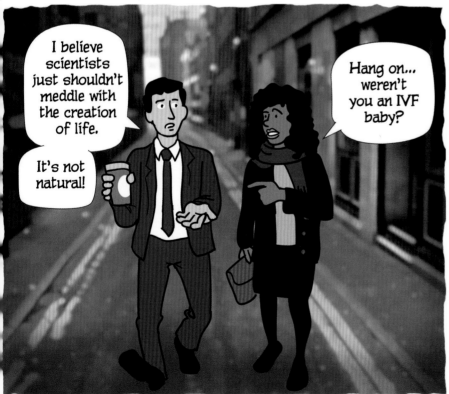

Science can only ever develop as fast and as far as society will allow. In 1978 people feared Louise Brown, the first 'test tube baby', would turn out to be Frankenstein's monster. She wasn't and now IVF treatment is routinely used to help couples to have children. Perhaps this generation is ready to accept that same procedure will be used to help couples have healthy children.

And of course those children should have the right to know how they were conceived if not by whom. Actually, the term 'third parent' seems a bit of a stretch. The donor will actually only be making a genetic contribution of 0.1 of one per cent.

Yes, the science is untested outside the lab and as with every development there is an element of risk. There is more work to be done. But this consultation is not about is it safe, it's asking is it right?

At its most basic emotional level, this is about saving 100 babies every year from disease. This is about saving women from having to bury their children, sometimes just months after they were born. Most mothers will tell you they would do anything, consider anything, pay anything to stop their children suffering, to stop them dying. This, then, is their hope.

"However you look at this procedure, this is genetic modification and it is an alteration of what is known as the germline"

While the consultation here is very specific, there is no doubt the ramifications of saying yes to the genetic modification of human beings is profound. Professor Lisa Jardine, the chair of the HFEA, is right when she says 'everyone in Britain should have a view on this'. It is too important an issue not to make your opinion heard – whether you agree with me or not.

Steve: Yes – we need to draw a line

As someone who has become a father in the past 15 months and is still full of the overwhelming wave of emotion that brings, I can completely understand the glimmer of hope that this procedure could offer to a relatively small number of people affected by these conditions.

It could transform lives and remove the threat of one of a host of devastating disorders being passed on by seemingly helpless parents to their unborn children. However, I am still wary that such a move would be too far in a direction that science and society would never be able to return from.

However you look at this procedure, this is genetic modification and it is an alteration of what is known as the germline. That change would be permanent and then passed down to future generations. If there were unforeseen medical problems from this technique, then they would be inherited not only by the child but also their descendants.

It is fiddling with the building blocks of how we are actually made. I would join the voices of the many experts who have quite rightly asked whether we have the right or maturity as a species to meddle with nature in this way.

"At its most basic emotional level, this is about saving 100 babies every year from disease. This is about saving women from having to bury their children"

The team leading the way with this research at the University of Newcastle claim the mitochondria is simply the battery of a cell and has no connection with deciding the characteristic. But bioethicists suggest that the true importance of the mitochondria genome is not fully understood by scientists so to dismiss it as simply the energy supply of a cell could be wrong or misleading. Do we really know enough about what we are playing around with here?

There is also the fundamental issue of how safe this procedure is. The team in Newcastle who have succeeded in creating the process in the lab says it will take three to five years to ensure that it is safe and there is no risk of disease. But are such processes ever safe? These are ultimately experimental techniques and there are numerous occasions in science where something which was thought to be safe turned out to be harmful.

What about the effects on the child itself? How will he or she feel to be born through such techniques, would they have a relationship with the donor of the egg? Would she have any rights as a donor? What about the effects on the parents? Although there are similar examples such as surrogate mothers, this is uncharted territory and passage through that territory has yet to be convincingly argued.

Ultimately, we have to put aside those emotions I referred to about the children and parents affected by this rare genetic hand of fate and look dispassionately at a scientific advance that may be one step too far down the ethical debate of how much power the human being has over being human.

Husband and wife pairing Steve and Zoe Vaughan share a background in journalism, an interest in current affairs and a passion for triathlons.

20 July 2012

⇨ The above information is reprinted with kind permission from MSN UK News. Please visit http://news.uk.msn.com for further information.

Sex selection

What is sex selection?

The term 'sex selection' is used to refer to various processes that allow you to choose the sex of an embryo.

In the UK sex selection is only allowed for medical reasons; for example, to avoid giving birth to children with a sex-linked genetic disorder like Duchenne muscular dystrophy. These diseases affect boys but not girls (girls may still 'carry' the gene for the disease but they will not suffer from it).

Is sex selection for me?

The only situation in which you should be advised to use sex selection is in the case of medical need, such as being at risk of passing on a known genetic disease that affects children of one sex only. In this case, it is acceptable to select the sex of an embryo so it will be unaffected by the disease.

How does sex selection work?

In the UK, pre-implantation genetic diagnosis (PGD) is currently the only method used in practice to choose the sex of the baby.

You may hear about the other methods listed:

⇨ Sperm sorting – this is where sperm are selected according to whether they carry male or female chromosomes.

A sample of the chosen sperm is then used to inseminate a woman or create IVF embryos in the lab. The only method of sperm sorting that is currently permitted in the UK is flow cytometry, which uses fluorescent dye to separate sperm carrying male chromosomes from those carrying female ones.

This method is not 100% reliable, so it is not used in practice.

⇨ Folklore and 'natural' methods such as the timing of intercourse to favour the conception of a child of a particular sex.

⇨ Selective abortion of foetuses that are shown by ultrasound to be the sex that is not wanted.

Since the changes to the EU law in July 2007, all clinics that offer sperm processing must be licensed by the HFEA and must only offer sex selection for medical reasons.

What are the risks of sex selection?

Most of the risks involved in sex selection treatment are similar to those for conventional in vitro fertilisation (IVF).

With sex selection, there is also the possibility that:

⇨ some embryos may be damaged by the process of testing

⇨ no embryos are suitable for transfer to the womb after sex selection (i.e. all embryos are of the sex being selected against)

⇨ flow cytometry is not 100% reliable, which is why it is not normally offered.

New genetic testing techniques

Some scientists are developing genetic tests that look for the specific genes that cause sex-linked disorders, such as Duchenne muscular dystrophy or Haemophilia A.

This means that you may be able to select male or female embryos that do not carry the gene for the disease, instead of just selecting against all male embryos.

⇨ The above information is reprinted with kind permission from the Human Fertilisation & Embryology Authority (HFEA). Please visit www.hfea.gov.uk for further information.

© HFEA 2013

Sex selection in the US is still legal. But what do the experts say?

High-tech sex-selection methods have stirred hot debate in the medical community. Some doctors think it's a great way to balance families, while others think we're heading down a slippery slope.

Mark Sauer, a fertility specialist and the program director at the Center for Women's Reproductive Care at Columbia University in New York, thinks that sex selection for family balancing is unethical and has no place in fertility treatments.

'I can't endorse the destruction of normal human embryos because they happened to be of the wrong sex,' he says.

Not all fertility doctors agree with Sauer. While the American Society for Reproductive Medicine officially opposes PGD for nonmedical reasons, it acknowledges that sex selection shouldn't be condemned in all cases and doesn't favour making it illegal.

Low-tech sex selection has not sparked the same controversy, probably because these methods are far from foolproof and the assumption is that couples practising them are investing less – both financially and emotionally – in their success. But do they work?

These techniques range from Shettles and Whelan to folk wisdom such as making love standing up and eating more meat if you want a boy, and eating lots of chocolate and having sex in the missionary position if you want a girl.

'I tell my patients that if they want to try low-tech methods, give them a go,' says Brian Acacio, a fertility specialist and medical director of the Sher Institutes of Reproductive Medicine (SIRM) in Los Angeles. 'They probably won't hurt, and there's a 50 per cent chance they'll work.'

Extract from babycenter.com. © BabyCenter L.L.C.

British couples flying to US for banned baby sex selection

Dozens of couples are flying to the US every year to choose the sex of their babies, a practice banned in Britain in 2009.

By Stephen Adams

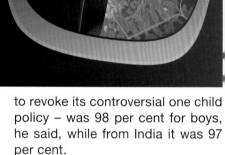

They are spending up to £30,000 a time on trips to New York, to guarantee a boy or a girl, according to a clinic.

Clients include senior British politicians, claims Dr Jeffrey Steinberg, the Cambridge-trained IVF specialist who heads the Fertility Institute's clinic in Manhattan.

Most of the couples already have two or more children, but only of one sex, and want either a boy or a girl to 'balance' the family, said Dr Steinberg.

Advances in IVF technology mean it is now possible to determine the sex of an embryo in the laboratory, before it is placed in the womb, with 100 per cent accuracy.

However, sex selection for social or 'family balancing' reasons was made illegal in the UK in October 2009, after the Government amended the Human Fertilisation and Embryology Act 1990.

Under the legislation, sex selection is only allowed for medical reasons, such as to avoid the risk of a child being born with a sex-linked genetic disorder like Duchenne muscular dystrophy, which only presents in boys. Similar laws exist in many other countries.

No such stipulations exist in many US states, with IVF clinics there seeking to capitalise on a growing desire among wealthy couples from around the world to design their families rather than leaving it to chance.

Speaking to *The Evening Standard*, Dr Steinberg, who trained alongside IVF pioneer Robert Edwards at the Bourn Hall Clinic in Cambridge, said 15 per cent of clients at the New York centre were British.

He said women first attended London clinics which were affiliated with Fertility Institutes, where they were given drugs to stimulate egg production, before flying to the US for the rest of the treatment.

Eggs are then collected, fertilised in the test tube, and then screened for genetic abnormalities and gender using a now well established technique called pre-implantation genetic diagnosis (PGD).

He claimed: 'I have had leading British politicians from the UK coming here, to this office, for services that are outlawed in the UK.'

Defending the right to offer sex selection, he said: 'The problem with all these countries where sex selection is not legal – Britain included – is that medicine and its financial arrangements are integrated into the Government.

'Once Government becomes involved in paying for everything, then Government starts making decisions about people's care.'

He admitted clients from some countries were almost exclusively interested in boys. Demand from China – currently under pressure to revoke its controversial one child policy – was 98 per cent for boys, he said, while from India it was 97 per cent.

Demand from the British was 'fairly evenly split, perhaps slightly favouring girls', he said.

He hoped his work would help prevent a small number of abortions in some countries, and argued it would have no effect on overall gender ratios because the figures were so small.

A spokesman for the Human Fertilisation and Embryology Authority (HFEA) said it had 'little or no remit' regarding British centres that provided preparatory care, such as those linked to Fertility Institutes.

'However, we do expect centres, whether referring patients abroad or recommending shared, cross-border care, to provide these patients with information about the consequences of having treatment outside the UK,' she said.

28 August 2012

⇨ The above information is reproduced with kind permission from *The Telegraph*. Please visit www.telegraph.co.uk for further information.

Saviour siblings

When a family has a child with a life-limiting condition, they can choose to 'tissue match' their new child to help its sibling:

⇨ They go to an IVF clinic to conceive their baby in a lab.

⇨ After three to four days, the embryo will have grown to 64 cells. It will fit on the head of a pin.

⇨ One cell is tested to see if there is a tissue match between the embryo and the family's sick child and, if necessary, to check that the embryo is free of genetic disorders.

⇨ If the embryo is a tissue match it can be implanted in its mother and allowed to continue to develop naturally.

⇨ Blood from the umbilical cord is collected after birth and can be used to treat the baby's sick sibling.

⇨ The family now has two healthy children!

This procedure is only allowed if there is no matching tissue donor in the family or on donor registries.

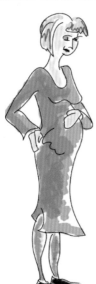

A handful of life-limiting conditions can now be treated using donated blood from umbilical cords (the link between a developing foetus and its placenta) or from bone marrow.

The cord blood or bone marrow contains stem cells that can develop into the specialised cells normally found in blood, which have a variety of functions needed for a healthy life, e.g. red blood cells transport oxygen around the body and different kinds of white blood cells are essential parts of our immune system.

The conditions that can be treated with these donated stem cells are all caused by a problem with one of the blood cell types, such as aplastic anaemia and severe combined immune deficiency (SCID).

If a matching donor can be found in a patient's family or on a bone marrow registry, this is the option that will be chosen for treatment of a patient. Unfortunately, only 25% to 35% of patients have someone in their family who is a match, and the chances of finding an unrelated matching donor is low and varies greatly with the ethnic origin of the patient.

Therefore, an alternative is to use IVF and embryo selection to have a second child who is a match for the affected child. This type of embryo testing (to select a tissue match) is only carried out if no matching donor exists.

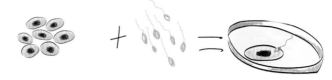

This 'saviour sibling' approach is tightly regulated by the HFEA and the welfare of the resulting child is a critical element of their decision-making. As stated by the Department of Health: 'Each application to the HFEA is considered on its own merits and the HFEA will grant a licence only where it is convinced that the child will be a valued member of the family and that tissue from the child is the only means of treating the older sibling.'

To date, licences have been granted to six families whose affected children have been cured of one of the following serious conditions: aplastic anaemia, Diamond-Blackfan anaemia and beta thalassaemia.

The new HFE Bill recognises that in future other tissues from tissue-matched siblings, such as cells from the umbilical cord itself, may be important for treating serious conditions, and it also explicitly allows for donation of bone marrow. The Bill outlaws tissue matching for whole organ donation. Licences for any saviour sibling procedure will continue to be considered on a case-by-case basis by the HFEA.

⇨ Illustrations by Rebecca Kent (rebeccajkent.com).

⇨ The above information is reprinted with kind permission from Genetic Alliance UK. Please visit www.geneticalliance.org.uk for further information.

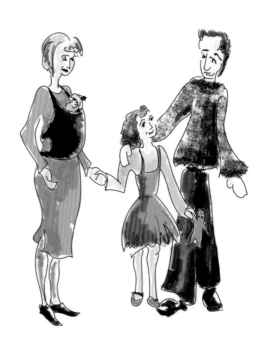

I prescribe one newborn baby brother

By Dave Vedage

Saviour siblings, as the name suggests, are children born to donate organs to and save the lives of their sibling. The benefits are obvious: the sibling would be treated, the newborn gets to help their relative and the family gets a new member.

However, the debate surrounding saviour siblings continues to rage on. The issue has also been reignited and brought to the attention of the wider public with the recent films *My Sister's Keeper* and *Never Let Me Go*.

Saviour siblings are possible by using in vitro fertilisation (IVF). By utilising HLA-typing and pre-implantation genetic diagnosis (PGD), it can be ensured that only zygotes compatible with the existing child are implanted and that the zygotes are free of the genetic disease. The first case occurred in 2000 in the USA. Newborn baby boy Adam Nash provided umbilical stem cells to his six-year-old sister, Molly, who was suffering from bone marrow failure secondary to Fanconi anaemia. In the United Kingdom, the Human Fertilisation and Embryology Authority has since ruled that it is lawful to use modern reproductive techniques to 'create' a saviour sibling.

Nonetheless, there still remains significant opposition. The basis of this argument is the idea that the child is merely a means to an end. This 'commodification' of human life is seemingly unnatural, but is it any less valid than other common reasons for wanting and conceiving a child, such as completing a family, saving a marriage, or providing an heir? Others argue that this is the start of a slippery slope that will lead to the creation of designer babies. There is quite a leap, however, between choosing a child with functioning bone marrow to one with blond hair, blue eyes and Brad Pitt's chin.

Then there is the strain that exists between the siblings, as they come to realise their unique and very unusual relationship. One child lives only because another one needed them to be born. This could engender feelings of worthlessness and resentment. Further psychological damage could be done if the elder child dies in spite of treatment, with the saviour sibling burdening themselves with the guilt of being unable to save their brother or sister.

However, that the parents are willing to conceive another child to protect the first suggests that they are highly committed to the wellbeing of their children and that they will value the second child for its own sake as well. Their birth may have served an instrumental purpose but they are almost invariably cherished for themselves. Furthermore, they may be considered beneficiaries of IVF, PGD and tissue typing, since were these techniques unavailable, they probably would not have been born.

Welfare is a fundamental principle. The main factor when deciding whether sibling saviours are ethically acceptable should be the degree of harm involved in the donation process. Though this can be balanced by the medical benefit to the older sibling, the harm to the saviour sibling does not necessarily depend on the severity of the affected child's condition. No medical intervention is without harm and if one must be performed within days or weeks of birth, this degree of harm must be weighed very carefully.

February 2012

⇨ The above information is reprinted with kind permission from the *Medical Student Newspaper*. The original article can be viewed at http://69.195.1 24.89/~themedn6/2013/04/23/i-prescribe-one-newborn-baby-brother/

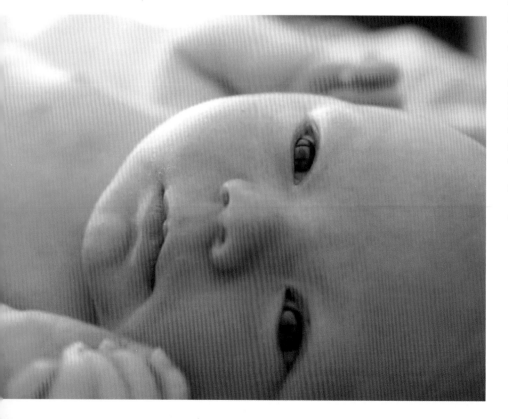

Should children be told they were donor-conceived?

Is the decision to tell children they were conceived using donor eggs or sperm a private matter for the family, or is this information so important that health and social care professionals should get involved?

The Nuffield Council on Bioethics has today launched a call for people's views on this and other ethical questions related to information about donor conception.

Many people support openness within families about donor conception, including organisations representing donor-conceived families and social workers, and the fertility regulator. The law was changed in 2005 so that donor-conceived children when they reach 18 can find out the identity of the donor and whether they have any half-brothers or sisters. But it is not clear how many families tell their children they were donor-conceived.[1]

Dr Rhona Knight, a GP and chair of the Nuffield Council inquiry, said: 'The law has changed to allow donor-conceived people to have more information about their donors, but many are unaware of their donor conception. We are interested in finding out why, and in hearing people's views on the responsibilities of families with regard to telling, as well as what kind of support they might need.'

The Council is also asking whether families should have access to more information about the medical and family history of the donor. Although donors are encouraged to provide full information about their family history, in practice the amount of information they make available can vary, or they may only become aware of important information after donation. People who have gone abroad for fertility treatment face even more difficulty in finding out about the history of the donor.

'The importance of information about the family history of the donor varies depending on the circumstances – what, or how much, is needed to ensure that donor-conceived children receive appropriate medical care during their lives?' asks Dr Knight. 'This can be a problem for health professionals too – if it comes to light that a donor has a genetic condition after a donation has taken place, clinics are often unsure what to do and who they can tell.'

There are further questions around whether donors should be entitled to receive more information about children born as a result of their donation. Donors are currently given very little information, unless the children decide to make contact when they turn 18.

In 2009, 1,756 children were born in the UK following donor conception treatment.[2]

The Council will use the views and evidence it gathers to inform an inquiry on the ethical issues that arise in connection with the disclosure of information about genetic origin in the context of families created using donor eggs, sperm or embryos, or surrogacy. The inquiry is being led by a Working Party that includes people with expertise in ethics, genetics, medicine, law, psychology and anthropology, as well as with direct personal and professional experience of donor conception issues. Over the next year, the Council will gather evidence and views from a wide range of people and organisations. The findings will be published in a report in spring 2013.

Questions that the Council is interested in include:

1. Should children always be told that they are donor-conceived? If so, why?

2. Who should decide whether, and if so when, to tell a child that they are donor-conceived? Is this a decision only the parents can take – or should anyone else be involved?

3. What information do the parents of donor-conceived children need about the donor to help them look after their child? Why?

4. What information about the donor do donor-conceived children need? Why?

5. What information (if any) might an egg, sperm or embryo donor want about a child born as a result of their donation? Why?

6. If a donor finds out later that they have a genetic condition, should they try to pass on this information to the child conceived with their egg/sperm?

7. What support might donors, donor-conceived children and parents of donor-conceived children need? Who do you think ought to provide it?

21 March 2012

⇨ The above information is reprinted with kind permission from Nuffield Council on Bioethics. Please visit www.nuffieldbioethics.org for further information.

1 Before the removal of donor anonymity in 2005, research found that 28 percent of parents of children conceived using donor sperm and 40 percent of parents of children conceived using donor eggs had told their child about their conception by the time they were seven. See: Readings J et al. (2011) Secrecy, disclosure and everything in between: decisions of parents of children conceived by donor insemination, egg donation and surrogacy. Reproductive BioMedicine Online 22, 485-495. More recent figures are not available.

2 www.hfea.gov.uk/donor-conception-births. html

Key facts

⇨ Not ovulating is the cause of infertility problems in three out of ten couples. (page 1)

⇨ Endometriosis causes about one in 20 cases of infertility. (page 2)

⇨ Male fertility problems occur in about two in ten cases. The most common reason for male infertility is a problem with sperm due to an unknown cause. The sperm may be reduced in number, less mobile or abnormal in form. (page 2)

⇨ Couples who do not conceive within three years still have a one in four chance of conceiving over the following year. (page 2)

⇨ Alcohol consumption and being overweight can both affect fertility. For the best chance at conceiving your BMI should be between 20 and 30. (page 3)

⇨ A woman's fertility does decline, and if you are over 35 you may find it more difficult to conceive than a 25-year-old. However, some women of that age, and older, conceive naturally without any problems. (page 5)

⇨ Women who smoke 20 cigarettes a day experience the menopause, on average, two years earlier than those who do not. (page 5)

⇨ The chances of a man getting his wife pregnant fall by seven per cent each year, between the ages of 41 and 45. (page 6)

⇨ In 2010, the percentage of IVF treatments that resulted in a birth were: 32.2% for women under the age of 35, 27.7% for women aged 35–37, 20.8% for women aged 38–39, 13.6% for women aged 40–42, 5% for women aged 43–44 and 1.9% for women over 44. (page 10)

⇨ In 2011, 41% of all IVF cycles performed were on women aged between 18 and 34. (page 12)

⇨ Studies now indicate that five million people have been born worldwide thanks to assisted reproductive technologies (ART). (page 13)

⇨ In the United States, approximately 120,000 children are adopted annually with nearly 50% being adopted by relatives. (page 14)

⇨ In England, in 2012, there were 37,050 children in local authority care. 3,450 children – 9% of the total number in care – were adopted during 2012. (page 15)

⇨ Conservative estimates show that more than 25,000 children are now being born through surrogates in India every year. The industry is worth approximately $2 billion. (page 20)

⇨ 50% of babies born through surrogates in India are 'commissioned' by overseas, mainly Western, couples. (page 20)

⇨ Guidelines now state that women aged between 40 and 42 who have not conceived after two years of regular unprotected intercourse, or 12 cycles of artificial insemination, should be offered one full cycle of IVF on the NHS. This only applies if they have never had IVF treatment before. (page 22)

⇨ In terms of fertility treatment, same-sex couples only account for 5% of NHS treatments. (page 24)

⇨ 45% of people surveyed by YouGov in February 2013 oppose the increase of the maximum age for IVF treatment from 39 to 42. 43% support the rise in age limit. (page 24)

⇨ The number of births for women aged 50 and older has risen 300% since 1997. (page 25)

⇨ 77.97% of respondents did not think that sex offenders should have the right to IVF treatment. 22.03% said they should. (page 28)

⇨ Around 6,000 adults in the UK are believed to be affected by mitochondrial diseases. (page 31)

⇨ Around one in 200 children are born each year with a form of mitochondrial disease. Some children have mild or no symptoms but others can be severely affected. (page 32)

Adoption

When a family becomes the legal guardians (adoptive parents) for a child who cannot be brought up by his or her biological parents. Couples who are infertile but wish to have a child look to adoption as an alternative. More recently, laws regarding adoption from overseas have become less strict.

ART/Artificial Reproductive Technology

'Fertility treatments': achieving pregnancy through artificial means.

Designer baby

A term coined by journalists, this refers to the use of gene therapy to determine what a baby will look like. There is a fear that this will lead to people using technology to select and 'customise' their baby before it's even born – selecting sex, height, appearance, eye/hair colour and possibly even IQ.

Donor/Donor rights

A donor is someone who donates either their eggs (female) or sperm (male) to be used in fertility treatments to help people who are unable to have children of their own. Donors used to remain completely anonymous, but in 2005 the law changed so that when donor-conceived children reach 18, they can find out the identity of the donor and whether they have any half-brothers or sisters (though this largely depends on whether they are ever told they are donor-conceived).

Eugenics

The belief that the human population can be improved through controlled breeding to increase the likelihood of more desirable heritable characteristics. For example, the Nazi party believed the Aryan race to be a master race and therefore their blonde hair and blue eyes were seen as superior characteristics.

Fertility/Infertility

According to doctors, infertility is when a couple are unable to become pregnant despite having regular, unprotected, sex for two years. There are a number of possible reasons for couples to be infertile. For example, male's low sperm count, damage to a female's fallopian tubes, etc.

Genetic testing

This refers to a technique called pre-implantation genetic diagnosis (PGD). This allows parents to test for serious genetically inherited conditions such Huntington's disease or cystic fibrosis. There is a fear that genetic

Glossary

testing will be misused (see *Designer baby*). However, it can be legally carried out if it is in the best interest for the embryo.

IVF (In vitro fertilisation)

IVF literally means 'fertilisation in glass', giving us the familiar term 'test tube baby'. IVF treatment is considered by couples who are having fertility problems and are not getting pregnant. Eggs are removed from the ovaries and fertilised with sperm in a laboratory dish before being placed in the woman's womb.

Saviour sibling

A child who is conceived because they will be a guaranteed tissue match for their sibling, who is affected with a fatal disease. Blood is collected from the saviour sibling's umbilical cord and can then be used to treat their unwell brother or sister. This is a very controversial procedure as some people feel it is wrong to conceive a child with the sole purpose of saving another. The procedure is only permitted if there are no matching tissue donors available anywhere else.

Surrogacy

When a couple who are unable to conceive naturally find another woman, known as the surrogate, to carry and give birth to their baby. Surrogacy is legal in the UK, but it is illegal to pay for the service. It is legal, however, to pay towards reasonable expenses such as medical costs.

Three-parent IVF

The process of creating a baby with three sets of DNA, rather than just the two – from the mother and father. This technique intends to help prevent inherited disorders as scientists can remove unhealthy mitochondria and replace them with healthy ones from a donor.

Assignments

1. Read the article *Infertility – a basic understanding* on page 1. Choose one of the common causes of infertility, such as polycystic ovary syndrome or endometriosis. Research your chosen cause of infertility and create a PowerPoint presentation that explains the science and statistics behind it. You should try to make your presentation engaging and easy-to-follow. Use pictures and diagrams to help you.

2. Age is an important factor when it comes to fertility and a lot of women do not realise they have a problem until they try to conceive. Create a campaign that will raise awareness of the things that younger women can do to protect their fertility. Your campaign could take the form of posters, television adverts or leaflets, but try to consider which one of these would appeal most to a younger demographic.

3. Design a leaflet that explains the risks and benefits of IVF treatment.

4. With a partner, discuss the emotional and physical effects that IVF can have on couples. Consider both female and the male perspective. Make some notes and feedback to your class.

5. Choose a country outside of the EU and investigate is laws surrounding fertility treatment, surrogacy and adoption. Write a short essay, summarising your findings.

6. Write a report summarising the debate surrounding three-parent IVF. What are the arguments for and against this method? Why is it so controversial? Try to include diagrams and/or statistics in your report.

7. Choose an illustration from this book and, in pairs, discuss what you think the artist was trying to portray with this image. Does the illustration work well with its accompanying article? If not, why not? How would you change it?

8. As a class, debate the following question: 'Should sex-offenders have the right to IVF treatment?'

9. Write a blog voicing your opinion about IVF treatment for women who are over the age of 40. Do you think treatment should be funded by the NHS? Do you think there should

be a cut-off-age at which IVF is not permitted? Maybe you think it's okay, as long as the woman is paying to have the treatment privately?

10. Mr and Mrs Turner both carry the gene for a genetic condition know as Sanfilippo syndrome. There is no cure for this disorder. They want to use IVF to select a healthy embryo and guarantee they have a child without Sanfilippo syndrome. In pairs, discuss the moral issues that are raised by this situation. Feedback and compare notes with the rest of your class.

11. Watch the film *My Sister's Keeper* (2009), or read the book of the same title by Jodi Picoult. Choose a character from the film/book and write a diary entry from their point of view, exploring their emotions and thoughts towards the concept of 'saviour siblings'.

12. Read the article *Should children be told they were donor-conceived?* on page 39. In small groups, think about questions 1–7 and make some notes on your thoughts. Feedback your ideas to the rest of your class.

13. Imagine there is a website called 'Surrogates R Us' where surrogate mothers and prospective parents can create profiles and contact one another. With a partner, design a prospective parent's profile. Your profile should include some personal information such as occupation, location, hobbies and beliefs. It should also include an advert specifying what you would like your surrogate to be like.

To take this further, consider whether you think it should be legal in the UK to advertise for surrogates/parents and create a bullet point list of pros and cons.

14. Sex selection is a controversial issue. Write a newspaper column in which you strongly agree or disagree with the process of sex selection. You should back-up your argument with further research such as statistics and facts.

15. Design a questionnaire that will investigate opinions surrounding IVF for same-sex couples. Try to distribute your questionnaire across a range of sexes and age-groups. Analyse your results and write a summary, including graphs.

16. Adoption is an alternative to IVF treatment and surrogacy. Create a website that promotes adoption as an alternative for people who are unable to have children.

17. Your friend, Ella, has decided she wants to act as a surrogate for her sister. Write an e-mail to Ella warning her of the legal and emotional implications of her decision.

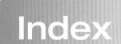

Acknowledgements

The publisher is grateful for permission to reproduce the following material.

While every care has been taken to trace and acknowledge copyright, the publisher tenders its apology for any accidental infringement or where copyright has proved untraceable. The publisher would be pleased to come to a suitable arrangement in any such case with the rightful owner.

Chapter 1: Infertility, IVF and alternatives

Infertility – a basic understanding © EMIS 2013, *Common fertility myths* © 2001-2013 Bounty (UK) Ltd, *Protect your fertility* © NHS Choices 2013, *Men have a ticking biological clock too, says study* © Martin Beckford/The Daily Telegraph, *Fertility treatment options* © HFEA 2013, *In vitro fertilisation* © NHS Choices 2013, *IVF treatment – roller coaster ride* © Compass Internet Ltd 2011, *Five million IVF babies born to date, study says* © BioNews 2013, *Adoption* © 2013 IVF-infertility.com, *Adoption UK's view on some key issues* © Adoption UK 2013, *Surrogacy* © HFEA 2013, *India's surrogate mothers are risking their lives. They urgently need protection* © Guardian News and Media Limited 2013.

Chapter 2: Reproductive ethics

Greater treatment options for women with fertility problems © NICE 2013, *Women over 40 should be offered IVF on the NHS, board suggests* © 2013 AOL (UK) Limited, *Columnist questions NHS funding IVF for over-40s* © The Christian Institute, *IVF mum, 57, now admits: 'I'm too old'* © BabyCenter L.L.C. 2013, *IVF: the older women who have become mothers* © Hannah Furness/The Daily Telegraph, *UK: anti-abortion group claims extending IVF to gay couples is 'social engineering'* © Pink News 2013, *Challenge to landmark ruling on sex offender's right to IVF (poll)* © 2013 AOL (UK) Limited, *'Three-parent IVF' could combat genetic disease* © Channel 4 2013, *Ethical committee finds IVF by three parents morally justified* © 2013 AOL (UK) Limited, *HFEA launches public consultation on 'three parent' IVF technique* © Family Law Week 2013, *The big question:*

are GM babies wrong? © Microsoft 2013, *Sex selection* © HFEA 2013, *Sex selection in the US is still legal. But what do the experts say?* © BabyCenter L.L.C., *British couples flying to US for banned baby sex selection* © Stephen Adams/The Daily Telegraph, *Saviour siblings* © Genetic Alliance UK 2013, *I prescribe one newborn baby brother* © Medical Student Newspaper 2013, *Should children be told they were donor-conceived?* © Nuffield Council on Bioethics 2013.

Illustrations:

Pages 5 & 23: Don Hatcher; pages 13 & 33: Angelo Madrid; pages 19 & 29: Simon Kneebone.

Images:

Page 2 © Emily Cahel, page 6 © h. koppdelaney, page 11 © AJU_photography, page 21 © Cara Acred, page 26 © Jackie Staines, page 36 © Hajnalka Ardai.

Additional acknowledgements:

Editorial on behalf of Independence Educational Publishers by Cara Acred.

With thanks to the Independence team: Mary Chapman, Sandra Dennis, Christina Hughes, Jackie Staines and Jan Sunderland.

Cara Acred

Cambridge

May 2013